HEALTH CARE DELIVERY IN INDIA

ACKNOWLEDGEMENT

I take this opportunity to thank all those who have been instrumental in helping me carry out this project. First, I would like to thank **GOD, the Almighty** for all the blessings he bestowed on me and for being with me in all my endeavours. The successful final outcome of this research required lots of guidance and assistance from many people and I am extremely fortunate to have such people who heled me complete my work.

I express my sincere thanks to **Dr PADMA K BHAT** (Professor and Head of the Department), for her valuable and timely advice, and guidance that has helped me in accomplishing this task.

With deep sense of gratitude, I thank my guide, **Dr PRASANNA KUMAR Y.S, Professor** for his patience and valuable guidance, unflinching support, keen surveillance, constructive inputs and constant help, which has been instrumental in moulding me as a professional and motivated me throughout this project.

I express my sincere thanks to **Dr JAYACHANDRA M Y**, Reader for his support, guidance, prompt advice, encouraging remarks and empowerment that helped me accomplish this task. I am extremely grateful for his kindness and acceptance.

I wish to express my warm and sincere thanks to, **Professor, Dr Aruna C.N, Professor, Dr Shweta Somasundara Y, Dr Anjan G, Dr Santhosh Kumar,** for their guidance and kind support that has been of great value for this study.

My heartfelt gratitude to my postgraduate colleagues, **Dr. Gyathiri R and Dr. Abhilasha S. Byalod,** and my seniors, **Dr. Subodh Kumar, Dr. Nigy Johnson, Dr. Karishma S Halageri, and Dr. Nayana M.** Department of Public Health Dentistry, Rajarajeswari Dental College and

Hospital for all the help and constant encouragement rendered during various stages of this project.

I would also like to thank the post graduate students and staff, **Department of**, Rajarajeswari Dental College and Hospital and patients for their valuable time and support.

My beloved parents **Mr. MURUGESAN P, Mrs. DHANALAKSHMI M,** the pillars of my life, thank you both for the unwavering love and faith, prayers and sacrifices for education and preparing me for my future life. I also thank My brother **Dr NAATCHI MUTHU P M,** for installing great strength and confidence in me and My sister-in-law **Dr ABENAYA** for constant support and motivation they give to keep me going. My special thanks to my dear friends **Dr AISHWARYA** for constant support and encouragement.

Finally, I would like to thank each individual who was important to the successful completion of this project. I would also like to express my apology towards those whom I could not thank personally.

Thank you one and all.

Dr ARUMUGAM P M

LIST OF ABBREVATIONS

(In alphabetical order)

ABP – Ayushman Bharath Program

ACA – Affordable Care Act

AHA – American Hospital Association

AIIMS – All India Institute of Medical Science

ANC – Anti Natal Check up

ANM – Auxiliary Nurse Midwife

ASHA – Accredited Social Health Activist

AWC – Anganwadi Centre

AWHs – Anganwadi Helpers

AWW – Anganwadi Workers

BCC – Behaviour Change Communication

BE – Budget Estimate

BMI – Basic Medical Insurance

BPHU – Block Public Health Unit

CAGR – Compound Annual Growth Rate

CHE – Country Current Health Expenditure

CHIP – Children's Health Insurance Program

CMS – Centres for Medicare and Medicaid Services

CNY – Chinese Yuan Renminbi

COVID – Corona Virus Infectious Disease

CPHC – Comprehensive Primary Health Care

DCI – Dental Council of India

DH – District Hospital

DOTS – Directly Observed Treatment Short course

EBMI – Employee Basic Medical Insurance

EHIC – European Health Insurance Card

ESI – Employees State Insurance

EU – European Union

FDI – Foreign Direct Investment

FPL – Federal Poverty Level

FRU – First Referral Unit

GBD – Global Burden of Disease

GCC – Gulf Cooperation Council

GDMO – General Duties Medical Officer

GDP – Gross Domestic Product

GPs – General Practitioners

GPHCF – Government Private Health Care Facility's

HMIS – Health Management Information System

HR – Human Resources

HWC-SHC – Health and Wellness Centres and Sub Health Centres

ICDS – Integrated Child Development Services

IDA – Indian Dental Association

IEC – Information, Education and Communication

IPHS – Indian Public Health Standards

IT – Information Technology

LMIC – Low Income and Middle-Income Countries

MAM – Moderate Acute Malnutrition

MAS – Mahila Arogya Samitis

MCO – Managed Care Organization

MHC – Maternal and Child Health

NCD – Non - Communicable Disease

NDMA – National Disaster Management Authority

NGO – Non – Governmental Organization

NHSA – National Health Security Administration

NHI – National Health Insurance

NHP – National Health Policy

NOHCP – National Oral Health Care Program

NRHM – National Rural Health Mission

NSHIF – National Social Health Insurance Fund

NUHM – National Urban Health Mission

OECD – Organization for Economic Cooperation and Development

OMI – Obligatory Medical Insurance

OOPE – Out of Pocket Expenditure

OPD – Out Patient Department

PHCs – Public Health Care Centres

PHC – Primary Health Centres

PHC – Primary Health Care

PMJAY – Pradhan Mantri Jan Arogya Yojana

PNC – Post Natal check up

PPP – Public Private Partnership

PRI – Panchayati Raj Institution

RBMI – Resident's Basic Medical Insurance

RCH – Reproductive and Child Health

RE – Revised Estimate

RTI – Reproductive Tract Infection

SAM – Severe Acute Malnutrition

SCI – Social Health Insurance

SDG – Sustainable Developmental Goal

SDH – Sub District Hospital

STI – Sexually Transmitted Infection

STEPs – STEP wise Approach to Surveillance

UAE – United Arab Emirates

ULB – Urban Local Bodies

UHC – Universal Health Coverage

UHWC – Urban Health and Wellness Centres

UK – United Kingdom

UNICEF – United Nation International Children's Emergency Fund

US – United States

USA – United States of America

USD – United States Dollar

VHI – Voluntary Healthcare Insurance

VHND – Village Health Nutrition Day

VHSNCs – Village Health Sanitation and Nutrition Committee

WHO – World Health Organization

HEALTH CARE DELIVERY

CONTENTS

SECTION 1

1. Introduction
2. Health Care Delivery
    - History of health care delivery
3. Health care delivery systems around the world – United States (US), Russia, United Arab Emirates (UAE), Africa, China, and Nordic countries.
4. Health care delivery in southeast Asian region
5. Health care delivery in India
    - Levels of health care delivery in India

SECTION 2

1. Oral health care delivery
2. Oral health care delivery in developed countries
3. Oral health care delivery in India
    - National oral health policy
4. Oral health care insurances in India

SECTION 3

1. Health insurance in India

SECTION 1

1. INTRODUCTION

We will begin with a conceptual overview of what we mean by a "healthcare system." Modern health care systems have many interrelated components, so it can be useful to try to reduce the complexity for a moment and recognize the fundamental human and institutional participants in health care [1]. Health service integration is seen by the World Health Organization (WHO) as an essential requirement to achieve Universal Health Coverage (UHC). According to WHO, an integrated health service delivery is defined as, an approach to strengthening people-centeredred health systems through the promotion of the comprehensive delivery of quality services across the life-course, designed according to the multidimensional needs of the population and the individual and delivered by a coordinated multidisciplinary team of providers working across settings and levels of care with feedback loops to continuously improve performance and to tackle upstream causes of ill health and to promote well-being through intersectoral and multisectoral actions [2].

Most healthcare interactions involve consumers, professionals and facilitating organizations. In this scheme, consumers seek healthcare, professionals provide the care, and the facilitating organizations perform a myriad of supporting administrative, regulatory and financing functions to support or control these healthcare encounters. Most components of the United States (US) health care system fall primarily into one of these categories [1].

The health care delivery system of today has undergone tremendous change, even over the relatively short period of the past decade. New and emerging technologies, including drugs, devices, procedures, tests, and imaging machinery, have changed patterns of care and sites where care is provided. Health care utilization also has evolved as the population's need for care has changed over time. Some factors that influence need include aging, sociodemographic population shifts, and changes in the prevalence and incidence of different diseases. As the prevalence of chronic conditions increases, for example, residential and community-based health-related services have emerged that are designed to minimize loss of function and to keep people out of institutional settings [3].

In 2004, health and medical voluntary organizations in India, led by the People's Health Movement, urged political parties to support the right to health noting that the constitution provided a basis for such a right without the operational framework in place to ensure universal access to public health services [4].

2. HEALTH CARE DELIVERY

The challenge that exists today in many countries is to reach the whole population with adequate health care services and to ensure their utilization. The "large hospital" which was chosen hitherto for the delivery of health services has failed in the sense that it serves only a small part of the population, that too, living within a small radius of the building and the services rendered are mostly curative in nature. Therefore, it has been aptly said that these large hospitals are more ivory towers of diseases than centres for the delivery of comprehensive health care services. Rising costs in the maintenance of these large hospitals and their failure to meet the total health needs of the community have led many countries to seek 'alternative' models of health care delivery with a view to provide health care services that are reasonably inexpensive, and have the basic essentials required by rural population. A number of models have been developed for the delivery of health care services. One of the simplest models is,

The INPUTS and OUTPUTS of health care status:

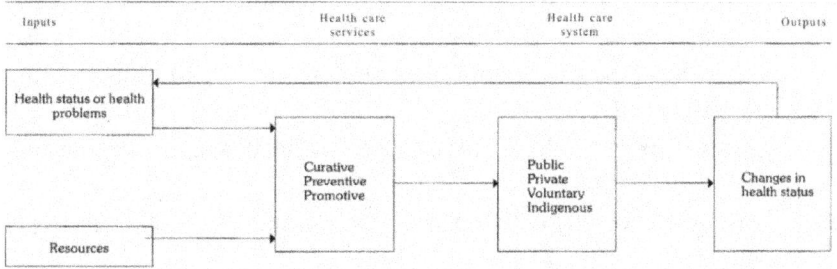

In actual practice the model is more detailed and complex. The INPUTS are the health status or health problems of the community; they represent the health needs and health demands of the community. Since resources are always limited to meet the many health needs, priorities have to be set. This envisages proper planning so that resources are not wasted. The HEALTH CARE SERVICES are designed to meet the health needs of the community through the use of available knowledge and resources. The services provided should be comprehensive and community-based. The resources must be distributed according to the needs of the community. The HEALTH CARE SYSTEM is intended to deliver the health care services; in other words, it constitutes the management sector, and involves organisational matters. The final outcome or the OUTPUT is the changed health status or improved health status of the community which is expressed in terms of lives saved, deaths averted, diseases prevented, cases treated, expectation of life prolonged, etc. Models such as these are being employed for improving health care services [5].

Health care systems are essential for improving and maintaining the health of the population of any country. Health systems are the result of the combined efforts of government agencies, institutions and resources with the main aim of improving the health of their people. Properly designed health systems have a strong preventive component which can detect possible illnesses through a combination of action and advice. An efficient health service can provide patients with advice on diseases that may be present and so facilitate treatment. It can also identify risk factors whose modification could reduce the incidence of disease and illness in the future and, further, advise on controlling such factors to contribute to maintaining a good quality of life [6] With its 3-tier public system of public health care centres (PHCs) in villages, district hospitals, and tertiary care hospitals, government expenditure in India has been shrinking, composing 0.9% of its gross domestic product (GDP) on health care, lower than the 2.8% of GDP expended by less developed countries. There has instead been an explosion in private health spending approaching 82% of all health spending. The paradox in health equity in India is exemplified by the poorest 20% receiving only 10% of available subsidies, whereas the richest 20% obtain 33% of them [7]. Over the past decade, both public and private organizations have made great strides in identifying causes of disease and disability, discovering treatments and cures, and working with practitioners to educate the public about how to reduce the incidence and prevalence of major diseases and the functional limitations and discomfort they may cause. Health care utilization also has evolved as the population's need for care has changed over time. Some factors that influence need include aging, sociodemographic population shifts, and changes in the prevalence and incidence of different diseases. As the prevalence of chronic conditions increases, for example, residential and community-based health-related services have emerged that are designed to minimize loss of function and to keep people out of institutional settings [3].

HISTORY OF HEALTHCARE:

The Indian healthcare scenario presents a spectrum of contrasting landscapes. At one end of the spectrum are the glitzy steel and glass structures delivering high tech Medicare to the well-heeled, mostly urban Indian. At the other end are the ramshackle outposts in the remote reaches of the "other India" trying desperately to live up to their identity as health subcentres, waiting to be transformed to shrines of health and wellness, a story which we will wait to see unfold. With the rapid pace of change currently being witnessed, this spectrum is likely to widen further, presenting even more complexity in the future. Our country began with a glorious tradition of public health, as seen in the references to the descriptions of the Indus valley civilization (5500–1300 BCE) which mention "Arogya" as reflecting "holistic well-being." The Chinese traveller Fa-Hien (tr.AD 399–414) takes this further, commenting on the excellent facilities for curative care at the time. Today, we are a country of 1,296,667,068 people (estimated as of this writing) who present an enormous diversity, and therefore, an enormous challenge to the healthcare delivery system. This brings into sharp focus the WHO theme of 2018, which calls for "universal health coverage- everyone, everywhere" [8].

Health is fundamental to national progress in any sphere. In terms of resources for economic development, nothing can be considered of higher importance than the health of the people. For the efficiency of industry and agriculture, the health of the worker is an essential consideration. However, the loss caused by morbidity is enormous. To this must be added the expenditure to the individual and the State in the provision of medical care. The causes of this low state of health are many including lack of a hygienic environment conducive to healthful living, low resistance to infections primarily due to poor nutrition, lack of safe water supply and of proper removal of human wastes, and most important, the lack of appropriate health care. These are serious impediments to progress [9].

Post-Independent India:

India became an independent nation in 1947 after remaining under foreign domination for more than 150 years. The economic, social, religious, and political exploitation during this period was beyond comprehension. On one side independence brought delight and joy but on the other hand it faced problems like population explosion, retarded economic development, mass illiteracy, and multilingual problems, etc. The Government of India set up the Planning Commission in 1950 to prepare a plan for the most effective and balanced utilization of the country's resources. In all plan periods, health had a separate allocation, but it always received a low priority. Health being a state subject led to every state having its own plan. However, the main thrust of Centre was to start the community development programme and national extension movement. The community development programme pledged itself towards self-help. The concept of democratic decentralization adopted by the government theoretically shifted the responsibility for health to the people themselves, through the Panchayatraj system. In actual practice it was a failure, except for the opening of 725 Primary Health Centres, and some effect on control of communicable disease. In course of time, when the government found that recommendations of Bhore Committee (1946) were too ambitious, it set up The Health Survey and Planning Committee, popularly known as Mudaliar Committee, in 1959.

This Committee was set up with the following aims:

1. To assess the progress in the field of medical relief and public health service since the submission of the Bhore Committee report.

2. To review the progress of First and Second Five Year Plans (Health Projects).

3. To formulate recommendations for the future plan of Health Development in the Country. The Health Survey and Planning Committee submitted its report in 1961.

This report was submitted some 15 years after the Bhore Committee, 10 years after the introduction of programmed systematic development in the form of Five-Year Plans. The result of systematic approach towards health care development programme has paid dividends in the field of control of epidemic diseases such as plague, cholera, malaria, and eradication of smallpox [10].

Study Group on Hospitals—1966:

After independence, under three Five Year Plans Rs 770 crores were spent but the results were not all that spectacular. This led the Ministry of Health and Family Planning, Government of India to set up the study group on hospitals in August, 1966. The study group was required to take into consideration the findings of previous committees that had examined different aspects of hospital administration, shift the material already available in those reports, and demarcate the fields to be further strengthened. Its recommendations were to be made with due regards to the financial position and the known insufficiency of manpower.

More specifically, the recommendations of the group were invited on the following:

1. The future pattern of development of hospital services at the regional, district, and peripheral levels in terms of size and facilities to be provided; the requirements of specialist hospital facilities, such as infectious diseases, tuberculosis, mental diseases, paediatrics, chronic and convalescent homes; and phased programme of development to achieve the recommended targets.

2. Measures required for integrated development of hospital services so that peripheral units like health centres, dispensaries, MCH centres work in close coordination with the hospital, which acts as the referral centre; specialist coverage of the peripheral units and referral hospitals by the teaching hospital in the region so that two or three districts have the medical college as a final referral centre.

3. Appropriate standards of staffing, drugs, diets, linen, etc., for hospitals of various sizes.

4. Provision of hospital pharmacies, central sterilization facilities and other services like proper kitchens, mortuaries, medical record system, sanitation, and security arrangement, etc.

5. Measures for the augmentation of resources available for medical care facilities, including those of pay clinics, system of graded charges for services rendered, health care, etc.

6. Facilities for family planning.

7. Any other matter relevant to the objectives and purpose of the study [10]

3. HEALTH CARE DELIVERY SYSTEM AROUND THE WORLD

UNITED STATES (US)

The US health care system was built mainly in the twentieth century, although the ideas and institutions upon which it was founded are as old as the country itself. The foundations still guide its development, which has consisted mainly of incremental infilling to cover various vulnerable populations. The system is complex and difficult to navigate, which provides opportunities for organized interests to wield influence [11].

The U.S. health care system is unique among advanced industrialized countries. The U.S. does not have a uniform health system, has no universal health care coverage, and only recently enacted legislation mandating healthcare coverage for almost everyone. Rather than operating a national health service, a single-payer national health insurance system, or a multi-payer universal health insurance fund, the U.S. health care system can best be described as a hybrid system. In 2014, 48 percent of U.S. health care spending came from private funds, with 28 percent coming from households and 20 percent coming from private businesses. The federal government accounted for 28 percent of spending while state and local governments accounted for 17 percent. Most health care, even if publicly financed, is delivered privately. In 2014, 283.2 million people in the U.S., 89.6 percent of the U.S. population had some type of health insurance, with 66 percent of workers covered by a private health insurance plan. Among the insured, 115.4 million people, 36.5 percent of the population, received coverage through the U.S. government in 2014 through Medicare (50.5 million),

Medicaid (61.65 million), and/or Veterans Administration or other military care (14.14 million) (people may be covered by more than one government plan). In 2014, nearly 32.9 million people in the U.S. had no health insurance [12].

The US health care delivery system differs from those of other developed countries in three notable ways: It relies on multiple sources of private financing, it covers less of the population, and it costs much more. In 2013, the USA spent the equivalent of $8713 per person on health compared to the OECD average of $3453 (Organisation for Economic Co-operation and Development [OECD] 2015). Total US health expenditures accounted for 16.4 % of gross domestic product (GDP) compared to the OECD average of 8.9 %. Fifty-two percent of expenditures were privately financed—by insurers, corporations, and consumers—in contrast to approximately one quarter across the OECD. Yet, more Americans (15.5 %) lacked coverage for a core set of services than residents of all other countries, except Greece where the rate was 21 %. In fact, most other OECD countries provided universal coverage [13].

Base (Pre-ACA) System:

There are seven main sources of health insurance coverage in the United States – Country in North America (USA) — employer-sponsored (ESI), individual direct purchase, Medicare, Medicaid and Children's Health Insurance Program (CHIP), the Veterans Health Administration (VHA), the military, and the Indian Health Service (IHS). The benefits provided by each differ—for example, Medicaid covers custodial care in nursing homes, but Medicare does not—so "dually eligible" individuals often draw from multiple sources to maximize their coverage. For each source, care is financed and delivered separately; however, most financers influence the delivery systems, the combination of providers, care settings, and benefits those beneficiaries utilize Centres for Medicare and Medicaid Services (CMS).

Of the seven sources, ESI and individual insurance are financed privately, although employers and employees receive public benefits (in the form of tax exemptions, as well as direct premium subsidies); the remaining five are publicly financed, though insured individuals might have to make contributions in the form of premiums, coinsurance, and/or co-payments. Health care services for veterans, military personnel and their families, and IHS beneficiaries are typically delivered by public employees in public facilities. Privately insured individuals and Medicaid, Medicaid, and CHIP beneficiaries typically receive physician and ancillary care from private providers and hospital and skilled nursing care from a mix of non-profit, for-profit, and public institutions. According to the AHA (2016), just under 60 % of hospitals are nongovernmental non-profit institutions, 20 % are for-profit, and 20 % are government-owned. In the last 3 decades of the twentieth century, mergers, takeovers, and purchases of public hospitals by private chains led to some market consolidation.

More and more, services covered by ESI and individual insurance, Medicare, and Medicaid are contracted through for-profit and non-profit managed care organizations (MCOs) that accept a set per member per month (capitation) payment for these services [11].

The Affordable Care Act (ACA):

The ACA was the most comprehensive piece of health care legislation in US history—its provisions filled ten titles and thousands of pages. It was also the most ambitious, as denoted by its first title—Quality, Affordable Health Care for All Americans. Nevertheless, its aim was not to transform the US health care system, but to reform it, as previous bills have attempted to do, by filling in gaps. It built upon the US's private health system by incentivizing expansions of private health care coverage and extending Medicaid/CHIP coverage to populations that markets will not serve.

The ACA further embedded the role of private actors. Specifically, the ACA:

- Required most US residents to have health insurance or pay a tax penalty (thus creating a bigger private insurance market)
- Required states to set up health insurance marketplaces so that their residents can buy insurance.
- Publicly subsidized low-income persons' purchase of individual coverage & Incentivized employers by penalizing them for not covering employees, particularly low-income employees, and providing small employers with tax credits.

- Required states to expand Medicaid to all nondisabled, nonaged persons with income below 138 % of the FPL.
- Required all insurers to provide essential health benefits, to include preventive services and prescription drugs, and private insurers to spend more of their dollars on them & Reformed or eliminated private insurance practices that limited access, such as imposing high deductibles.
- Required states and insurers to provide assistance to consumers in navigating the system [11].

Common Methods to Lower Health Care Costs:

By taking an international perspective and looking to other advanced industrialized countries with nearly full coverage, much can be learned. While methods range widely, other OECD countries generally have more effective and equitable health care systems that control health care costs and protect vulnerable segments of the population from falling through the cracks.

Among the OECD countries and other advanced industrialized countries, there are three main types of health insurance programs:

- A national health service, where medical services are delivered via government-salaried physicians, in hospitals and clinics that are publicly owned and operated—financed by the government through tax payments. There are some private doctors but they have specific regulations on their medical practice and collect their fees from the government. The U.K., Spain, and New Zealand employ such a system.
- A national health insurance system, or single-payer system, in which a single government entity acts as the administrator to collect all health care fees, and

pay out all health care costs. Medical services are publicly financed but not publicly provided. Canada, Denmark, Taiwan, and Sweden have single-payer systems.

- A multi-payer health insurance system, or all-payer system, which provides universal health insurance via "sickness funds," used to pay physicians and hospitals at uniform rates, thus eliminating the administrative costs for billing. This method is used in Germany, Japan, and France.

A universal mandate for health care coverage defines these systems. Such a mandate eliminates the issue of paying the higher costs of the uninsured, especially for emergency services due to lack of preventative care. Other methods for reducing costs may include:

- Funding health care costs in relation to income rather than risk or people's medical history.

- Negotiating the price of prescription drugs and bulk purchasing of prescription medications and durable medical equipment is a method used in other countries for lowering costs. This has been effectively used by the U.S. Department of Veterans Affairs, Medicaid, and Health Management Organizations in the U.S. Yet, it has been prohibited by law from traditional Medicare. Savings of up to five percent of total health care expenditures could result from the full adoption of these practices [12].

Quality of U.S. Health Care in an International Context:

U.S. health care specialists are among the best in the world. However, treatment in the U.S. is inequitable, overspecialized, and neglects primary and preventative care. The end result of the U.S. approach to health care is poorer health in comparison to other advanced industrialized nations. According to the Commonwealth Fund Commission, in a 2014 comparison with Australia,

Canada, France, Germany, the Netherlands, New Zealand, Norway, Sweden, Switzerland, the U.K., the U.S. ranked last overall. In terms of quality of care, the U.S. ranked fifth, but came in last place in efficiency, equity, and healthiness of citizens' lives. Comparing other health care indicators in an international context underscores the dysfunction of the U.S. health care system [12].

RUSSIA

When the former Soviet Union fell apart in 1991, the new Russian Federation that came into being faced a major health crisis that became even worse over the next few years. In the mid-1960s, ironically just as the Soviet Union reached its highest point of economic development in relation to the West, life expectancy began a downward trend, largely brought on by rising mortality from heart disease among middle-aged working-class males. Between 1965 and 1980, male life expectancy declined from 64.0 years to 61.4 years for reasons that were at that time unexplained. By 1987, however, the average number of years lived by Russian men improved to 64.9 – the highest ever. Russian demographers credit this brief rise in male longevity to Premier Mikhail Gorbachev's anti-alcohol campaign in the mid-1980s, which significantly curtailed both the production and the consumption of vodka. With the collapse of the Soviet Union and the decline of Russia's standard of living in the 1990s, the decrease in life expectancy for both men and women accelerated. In 1994 longevity for men fell to a modern low of 57.6 years, and that for women to 71.2 years – only 0.1 years more than in 1965. Obviously, there was a health crisis in Russian society affecting both men and women that neither the new nor the old health care delivery system had been able to deal with.

FORMER SOVIET HEALTH CARE SYSTEM:

Prior to the collapse of communism, the health care delivery systems in the former Soviet Union and Eastern Europe were philosophically guided by Marxist-Leninist programs for reshaping capitalism into socialism. The ultimate goal was the establishment of a classless society, featuring an end to class exploitation, private property, worker alienation, and economic scarcity. The Soviet state established in the aftermath of the 1917 Revolution nevertheless faced serious health problems, including large-scale epidemics and famine. More out of practical than theoretical necessity, the Soviet government mandated that health care would be the responsibility of the state, provided without direct cost to the user, and controlled by a central authority; that worker would be given priority for care; and that the emphasis would be on preventive care [14].

Overview of Russia's Healthcare System:

Since 1996, Russia's constitution has provided citizens and residents with the right to free healthcare. This is provided by the state through the Federal Compulsory Medical Insurance Fund (also called the OMI or Obligatory Medical Insurance). It is funded through payroll and employer contributions. The Russian Ministry of Health oversees the system and its two million employees. Federal regions, such as Moscow, also have their own departments of health that oversee local administration.

Overall, OMI based care is comprehensive. It covers the cost of inpatient care, all procedures that require an overnight stay at the hospital, chronic conditions, maternal and new-born care, vaccinations, and more.

Like many countries, public hospitals in Russia struggle with long wait times and overcrowding. Unlike others, sometimes this reaches extremes and has a significant impact on the quality-of-care patients receive.

Compounding the problem is the fact that public hospitals are few and far between outside of large cities. Patients sometimes feel they're stuck between being in a very crowded hospital or having no hospital at all.

The bottom line is that Russians aren't happy. According to a 2016 survey by Moscow-based polling agency Levada Centre, only a paltry 2% of Russians reported being proud of their healthcare system. Some of the most alarming complaints include filthy hospitals, crumbling buildings, and even doctors and paramedics working while intoxicated [15].

Access of healthcare in Russia:

Every Russian citizen and resident receive free public healthcare under the Russian healthcare system via Obligatory Medical Insurance (OMI).

Foreign residents in Russia, both permanent and temporary, can access public healthcare through OMI. Many expat residents are also covered by voluntary healthcare insurance (VHI) which is supplementary insurance usually offered through employers.

Unemployed foreign citizens with a residence permit may eligible for an OMI policy under certain conditions; you will need to check via a medical insurance company that subscribes to the Russian healthcare system.

As of January 2016, the previous reciprocal healthcare agreement between the UK and Russia is no longer in effect, meaning that visitors to Russia from the UK need to take out private medical insurance. Other EU residents who carry a European Health Insurance Card (EHIC) should check with their home government whether they can access Russian healthcare before coming to Russia.

For non-EU citizens, you must check if your home country has a reciprocal healthcare agreement with Russia. Otherwise, you will typically need to show proof of healthcare coverage when applying for a Russian visa.

Costs of healthcare in Russia:

Russia spent 5.27% of its annual GDP on healthcare in 2016. However, this is below the current global average of around 10%. It is also lower than all EU countries except Romania.

Employers finance OMI through contributions. Once you begin working in Russia, your employer will pay around 2–3% of your salary into a social tax; a percentage of which is paid into a national Russian healthcare fund. Once an employer pays for this compulsory medical insurance, you have the right to free medical assistance from public Russian healthcare clinics.

Those who cannot contribute to OMI due to not working (e.g., unemployed, pensioners, children, those too ill to work) can still access free basic healthcare [15].

Challenges and Changes:

Russia's public healthcare system is struggling to keep pace with an aging population, aging infrastructure, and challenging political history. At the end of the Soviet Union, Russian healthcare was a mix of state of private systems, with nearly four times the doctors and hospital beds per capita. A period of funding cuts devastated the public system and gave the private sector space to grow. Gradually, things turned the other way and by 2013, public healthcare allotments per person increased tenfold. Sadly, this period of growth was short-lived and Russia's financial crisis of 2014 brought drastic cuts once again. As such, there hasn't been a sustained period of growth and investment that has allowed the public healthcare system to thrive [16].

Health insurance in Russia:

When you start working in Russia, your employer will register you for OMI and start making monthly contributions. Many employers also offer VHI coverage as part of their benefits package. This covers some treatments not included in OMI, such as dental care and some outpatient treatments.

Individuals in Russia can also take out separate private health insurance plans. Private insurance entitles you to the full range of healthcare services. With private insurance, you generally have to pay upfront and claim reimbursement from your insurance company.

Some insurance providers require pre-authorization, meaning that you must contact your insurance company before using medical services in Russia [16]

CHINA

The healthcare security system is an important institutional arrangement for reducing people's medical burden, improving people's well-being, and therefore maintaining social harmony and stability in China.

<u>The composition, coverage, and operational trend of China's national medical security system:</u>

The national medical security system in China is a multilevel system, with the Basic Medical Insurance (BMI) as the pillar and medical aid as the backup, and commercial health insurance, charitable donations, and medical mutual aid activities as supplementary services. The BMI system serves two groups of people: employees and residents. Employees are enrolled in the employee basic medical insurance (EBMI) program, and non-working residents are enrolled in the resident's basic medical insurance (RBMI) program. After being established in 2018, the National

Healthcare Security Administration (NHSA) has continued to improve the national medical insurance system so that RBMI can be better integrated. As of September 2020, more than 1.35 billion people (over 95% of China's population) are covered by one of the BMI programs, making it the world's largest healthcare security network. Among those covered, 337 million are covered by the EBMI, and 1.014 billion people are covered by the RBMI. The medical insurance fund is sustainable and growing. In 2019, the revenue of the national basic medical insurance fund (including maternity insurance) was CNY ¥2.44 trillion, and the expenditure was CNY ¥2.09 trillion. Medical aid ensures all citizens have fair access to basic medical services by supporting the section of the low-income populace to participate in the BMI by subsidizing the medical expenses that they cannot afford. Since 2018, medical aid has benefited 480 million low-income citizens, helped reduce their medical burden by approximately CNY

¥330 billion, implemented targeted poverty reduction measures for 10 million people in need who were impoverished due to illnesses, and ensured their basic medical security. Various social forces in the market also actively participate in supplementing the medical security system and have become an important element of the multilevel medical insurance system [17].

Characteristics and advantages of China's healthcare security system:

The Chinese government has always regarded people's health and life safety as its basic responsibility, by providing the BMI as a public good for all Chinese citizens. However, a deficit in coverage still exists between China and other countries with developed social security systems. The proportion of total medical insurance financing is about 2.5% of China's GDP, which is not high, but it is generally compatible with the per capita GDP of US $10,000 in China.

- Provide more. For one, government funding should be increased. From 2007 to 2019, government funding for medical security increased from CNY ¥91.3 billion CNY ¥800 billion, and the proportion of government spending on medical insurance increased from 1.87% to 3.50%. In 2020, the government subsidy for resident medical security reached CNY ¥550 per person.
- Stay within economic capabilities. To ensure the sustainable balance of the fund, financial overcommitment should be avoided, and the planning should be informed by the current level of economic development. The fund should meet the basic needs of people, but it should avoid becoming a welfare fund.
- Reinforcing the administration of the security system.

a) First, a nationally organized volume-based procurement and use of drug standard should be established. A total of 112 types of drugs were procured by China in three batches, with the costs decreasing by an average of 54%, which saved CNY ¥53.9 billion annually.

b) Second, the catalogue of medicines covered by the national health security system shou7ld be dynamically adjusted. Some obsolete drugs have been removed from the catalogue to make room for drugs with more clinical value.

c) Third, a reformation of medical insurance payment methods needs to be steadily implemented. In China, 97.5% of the local administrations have capped the total regional expense of medical insurance, and more than 30 pilot cities have launched diagnosis-related group payment systems.

d) Fourth, medical organizations should be strictly supervised and unlawful practices should be heavily penalized. In the past 2 years, 330,000 unlawful organizations were suspended, and CNY ¥12.56 billion in funds were retrieved.

In 2019, 69 inspection teams were sent to 30 provinces across the country to conduct unannounced field inspections, and CNY ¥2.232 billion in illegal funds were found [17].

<u>Building a multilevel medical security system to reinforce support capabilities:</u>

In recent years, China's commercial health insurance premium income has developed rapidly at an annual growth rate of 30%. In 2019, the premium income of commercial health insurance was CNY ¥706.6 billion, which represented a year-on-year increase of 29.7% [18]

To meet people's growing needs of health care in the new era, the government proposes to strengthen the triple security system, which includes basic medical insurance, critical illness insurance, and medical aid, and promote various complementary medical insurance programs for major and critical diseases. The development of commercial health insurance will be accelerated, more health insurance products will be offered, the individual income tax policies for commercial health insurance will be applied in a more effective way, and the scope of insurance products will be expanded [19].

<u>Seizing opportunities, meeting challenges, and promoting the high-quality development of medical security:</u>

The year 2020 is the final year of 13th Five-Year Plan, and it is also the year to lay a good foundation for the 14th Five-

Year Plan. Standing at this critical juncture, it is necessary to have a clear understanding of the challenges faced by health security. The demographics of the Chinese population poses serious challenges to the sustainability of the fund. The number of people over the age of 60 will exceed 300 million people at the end of the 14th Five-Year Plan, and the ratio of employees to retirees will continue to decline. Another serious challenge is that communicable diseases and chronic diseases pose a "double burden" on China's medical insurance funds. There is still a gap between the healthcare security support and the medical expectations of citizens. Medical security is highly relevant to the vital interests of the Chinese people as a whole. During the 14th Five-Year Plan period, the government will continue to promote the integrity of the multilevel medical security and guide the coordinated development of medical security, treatment, and medicine, so that the people can have more clear and accountable expectations for their health security and a greater sense of gain, healthy security and happiness in turn [17].

THE UNITED ARAB EMIRATES AND SAUDI ARABIA

Healthcare is a key priority for the governments of the UAE and Saudi Arabia, in part to address the changing needs of their populations – including the rise in non-communicable diseases like diabetes, and cancer. Since the discovery of petroleum in Saudi Arabia in 1938, and 20 years later in the UAE, both countries have developed into modern states with a high standard of living. Currently, about 50% of Saudi Arabia's GDP comes from oil and gas, compared with 30% in the UAE. As the world moves away from fossil fuels and towards more renewable energy sources, both countries have sought to shift their heavy reliance on oil to more sustainable revenue streams, including by building world-class healthcare systems that will attract investors, providers, manufacturers and medical tourists from around the globe. The visions for these systems are ambitious: entire cities devoted to health and well-being; futuristic facilities; an increase in remote care; and world-class research centres, all using the latest technology and artificial intelligence to offer unparalleled treatment and services. Expats from developed countries and Saudi and Emirati nationals all expect first-rate standards of care and want to be able to access specialist care without returning home or travelling abroad, as they often needed to do in the 90s and early 2000s, when Gulf Cooperation Council (GCC) countries lacked expertise in certain fields.

I. THE UAE:

The UAE's healthcare system has come a long way since its early days nearly 80 years ago. In 1943, the country's first healthcare centre was opened in Dubai, followed by its first hospital in the early 1950s. Nearly two decades later, the Ministry of Health was established. Today, healthcare in the UAE has evolved into a well-established network of players and services, with a system offering free healthcare to all UAE citizens, as well as private options for citizens and foreign residents. Let's delve deeper into the demographics of the country, the infrastructure of its healthcare system, and its most prevalent health issues.

With 10 million inhabitants, the UAE has the second-highest population in the GCC after Saudi Arabia. Unlike other countries in the region, the vast majority of the UAE's population (90%) is comprised of expats. More than 85% of inhabitants lives in urban areas, and 98% of those reside in the two largest emirates (Dubai and Abu Dhabi), where medical insurance coverage is mandatory.

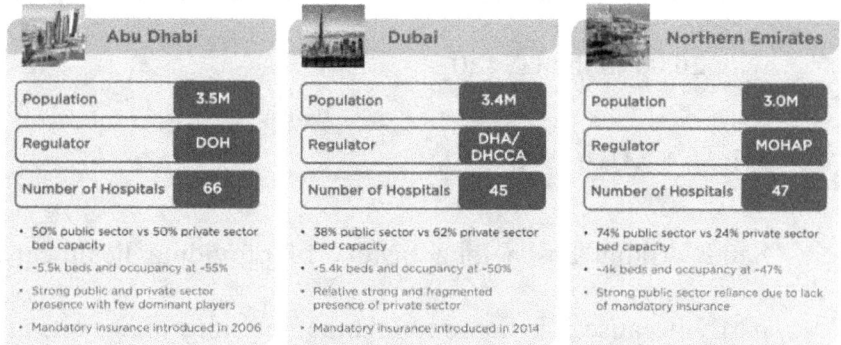

Source: Benhameurlaine, K. Ruiz, S. Nahlus, R. (2021) UAE Health Sector Pulse. Alvarez & Marsal.

Although the UAE intends to expand its healthcare system, the current infrastructure is relatively 4 robust, with 158 hospitals and 15,000 beds across the country. Over the past ten years, the number of hospitals has grown steadily – by 6.2% – and, while the split between public and private hospitals varies by emirate, Abu Dhabi and Dubai have the largest number of private 5 hospitals. Overall, the bed capacity in the public sector is higher than in the private sector, and the steady increase in the number of hospitals has led to a competitive healthcare provider 6 market. The ratio of physicians per 10,000 people is 25.3, compared with 26.04 in the US [20].

II. SAUDI ARABIA:

Saudi Arabia has a long history of providing healthcare, partly because it is home to Islamic holy pilgrimage sites to which millions of Muslims from around the world flock each year. These mass events have required significant preventative and responsive measures from the kingdom's healthcare system to ensure the safety of the pilgrims. This includes managing issues associated 13 with mass gatherings, such as the potential spread of diseases. Modern healthcare in the country was established by royal decree in the holy city of Mecca in 1925, and a quarter of a century later, the Ministry of Health was established. Today, Saudi Arabia offers free healthcare to all its citizens, alongside private healthcare options.

Saudi Arabia is the most populous country in the GCC, with 35 million people – the population is expected to grow to 39 million by 2030. The median age is 32 years, with an average life expectancy of 76 years. Saudi nationals make up 61.2% of the population. The size of the elderly population is growing, with the number of people aged 60 and older expected to more than double by 2030, from 1.8 million (5.5%) to 4.9 million (11.1%). This will affect the healthcare system as more people require geriatric services like long-term care and 14 rehabilitations.

Healthcare infrastructure:

There are 504 hospitals in Saudi Arabia, with nearly 78,600 hospital beds – an increase of around 11% since 2016. More opportunities for the private sector will emerge over the next few years, as estimates suggest that nearly 20,000 additional beds will be needed by 2035. In 2019, the highest number of private hospital beds was in the capital Riyadh (25%), followed 15 by Jeddah (24%), with the overall market share of private hospitals in Saudi Arabia expected to reach 30% in the next ten years. By 2030, 295 hospitals and 2,259 healthcare centres are expected to be privatised.

Countrywide Current Health Expenditure (CHE)
Healthcare Expenditure, Average of 2015-2019

Coutntry	GDP per capita on health in $	Goverment contribution to total healthcare expenditure
KSA	1,095	66%
UAE	1,358	71%
Bahrain	1,120	58%
Oman	590	88%
Qatar	1,650	80%
Kuwait	1,530	88%
World	1,061	60%

Source: https://countryeconomy.com/government/expenditure/health/

UAE's Vision 2021 and 2071:

The UAE has the ambitious goal of becoming the best country in the world and recognises that its population must be fit and healthy to achieve this. In 2014, the country launched its Vision 2021 strategy (extended until 2022 due to COVID-19), with the aim of building a world-class healthcare system.

Its key objectives include:

- Having all hospitals accredited according to national and international quality standards
- Reducing cancer and diseases like diabetes and cardiovascular disease
- Reducing the prevalence of smoking
- Increasing the healthcare system's readiness to deal with epidemics
- Increasing the number of physicians and nurses per 1,000 people

While Vision 2021 is still underway, the government has reaffirmed its commitment to the healthcare sector in its recently launched Vision 2071 plan. In addition to previous goals, Vision 2071 will also focus on efforts to improve access to healthcare through e-health and smart health, and to become a top destination for medical tourism [20].

Within these goals there are specific aims to modernise and advance the current healthcare system, including:

- Using AI to minimise chronic and dangerous diseases
- Adopting plans and strategies in the field of genomic medicine
- Developing personalised genome medications for patients
- Promoting medical tourism
- Focusing on robotic healthcare
- Enhancing telemedicine services
- Providing smart medical solutions 24/7
- Encouraging neuroscience research

In order to achieve the aims of both Visions, the UAE government is underpinning its efforts with significant investments. For example, in late 2020, USD 1.3bn (6.89% of the total budget) was allocated to healthcare spending for 2021. There has also been significant private investment in healthcare facilities and services.

<u>Saudi Arabia's Vision 2030:</u>

- The Ministry of Health is estimated to have spent nearly USD 71bn on healthcare by the end of 2020, with a compound annual growth rate (CAGR) of 12.3%, to reach its Vision 2030 goals. These include:
    - Increasing private healthcare spending from 25% to 35% of overall healthcare spending
    - Increasing the number of hospitals that are internationally accredited
    - Reducing the prevalence of smoking throughout the country
    - Increasing innovations in digital healthcare

- Spending more than USD 66bn on healthcare infrastructure
- Lowering the number of deaths from non-communicable diseases
- Achieving a 3% decrease in obesity and a 10% decrease in diabetes rates

There will be a particular focus on privatisation to transform the healthcare system. The government aims to reduce its own role from provider to regulator, and to increase private participation – a goal boosted by new regulations introduced in 2017. These have allowed foreign businesses to hold up to 100% ownership of companies in the sector, and mandatory health insurance for all expatriates is already in place.

By 2030, the government aims to increase the private sector's contribution to GDP from 40% to 60%, including through the privatisation of one of its medical cities.

It also aims to expand public-private partnership (PPP) healthcare delivery models, and to transform digital information systems and IT capabilities with a USD 1.5bn budget.

Healthcare will get a boost in the country from giga-projects like NEOM – a new futuristic city worth USD 500bn that will span over 10,000 square miles and include a Health Tech hub and medical research centres [20].

AFRICA

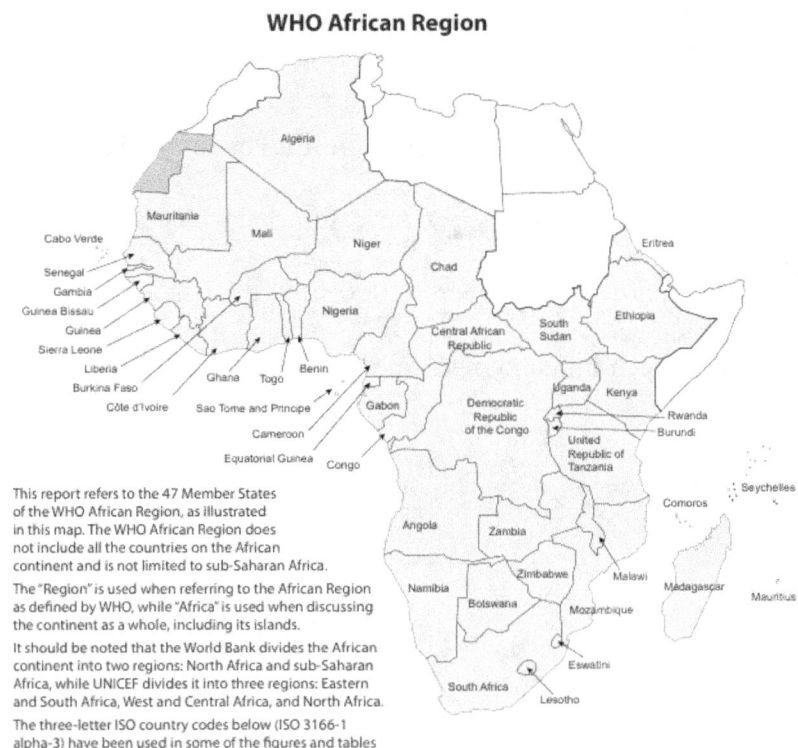

WHO African Region

This report refers to the 47 Member States of the WHO African Region, as illustrated in this map. The WHO African Region does not include all the countries on the African continent and is not limited to sub-Saharan Africa.

The "Region" is used when referring to the African Region as defined by WHO, while "Africa" is used when discussing the continent as a whole, including its islands.

It should be noted that the World Bank divides the African continent into two regions: North Africa and sub-Saharan Africa, while UNICEF divides it into three regions: Eastern and South Africa, West and Central Africa, and North Africa.

The three-letter ISO country codes below (ISO 3166-1 alpha-3) have been used in some of the figures and tables of the report for conciseness.

The overall average healthy life expectancy is on an increasing trend in the African Region, from 50.9 years to 53.8 years for the period 2012– 2015. It is trend is also seen with the median healthy life expectancy, which has increased from 50.1 to 53.6 years between 2012 and 2015. This suggests an improving trend in overall health and well-being of the persons living in the Region. Four countries – Algeria, Cabo Verde, Mauritius and the Seychelles – have a significantly better life expectancy compared to the other countries, and nine other countries have a healthy life expectancy under 50 years, representing a large loss in healthy life. There has been a reduction in the range of healthy life expectancy across countries in the Region in the past 5 years, which went from 27.5 to 22 years. This suggests a reduction of differences between countries of the region, although the differences are still significant. The levels of healthy life in the African Region remain much lower than the rest of the world. The Region is the only WHO region with a healthy life expectancy under 60 (52.3 years as compared to the next lowest, the Eastern Mediterranean Region, at 60.1 years). The African Region has a 16.4 - year gap in healthy life as compared to the Western Pacific Region, the best performing region globally, representing a major disparity for its population.

Risk factors influencing healthy life in the African Region:

Risk factors influencing healthy life remain a key area of concern in the African Region, as they are associated with fuelling the disease burden patterns observed. The Global action plan for the prevention and control of NCDs (2013–2020)15 recommends that countries focus on addressing four conditions (chronic respiratory disease, cardiovascular disease, cancer and diabetes) through four risk factors (alcohol abuse, insufficient physical activity, unhealthy diets and tobacco use). At present, a person in the African Region aged between 30 and 70 years has a 20.7% chance of dying from one of these major NCDs, a probability consistent with the global pattern or 19.4%. The lowest probability of dying from these NCDs is seen in the Region of the Americas (15.4%) and the European Region (18.4%), which may be a function of the highly specialized services available to populations in some countries of these regions. Efforts to make available highly specialized services responding to these NCDs can therefore bear fruit. There is a significant risk associated with each of the four risk factors contributing to this level of mortality: 1. alcohol consumption (6.3 L of pure alcohol consumption per capita per year); 2. insufficient physical activity (82.3% and 87.9% inactivity amongst male and female adolescents respectively); 3. unhealthy diets (7.7% and 15.1% children and adolescents' obesity respectively); and 4. tobacco use (24.2% and 2.4% tobacco use amongst 15 years old male and females respectively). Insufficient physical activity and unhealthy diet are significantly higher amongst females, while use of tobacco products is higher amongst males. Furthermore, there is evidence from the WHO STEP wise approach to surveillance (STEPs) surveys in countries of the Region that some of the risk factors – particularly tobacco use – are increasing disproportionately more amongst females than males, especially in adolescents. These findings suggest a need for strategies focused on different sexes and age groups [21]

In terms of health care, governments face a number of challenges, including lack of funds and poor infrastructure. This is compounded by epidemics, poverty and the brain drain of homegrown doctors moving abroad, in search of higher wages and a better standard of living. Varying wildly from country to country and region to region, public health care does exist but most expats will want to use the private sector (often based in large cities and major tourist locations) or have the **international health insurance** and funds to be **evacuated to another country.**

Nigeria:

While Nigeria has a public health service financed through a national insurance scheme, newcomers to the country might want to consider their own private medical insurance, use private health care facilities, and make sure they are covered for repatriation (in the event of death) or medical evacuation to another better-equipped country, if necessary. Public health care is improving, but it faces a number of difficulties including a low ratio of doctors at only 1 per 2,000 inhabitants (low on a global scale but higher than most of its African neighbours) and an infrastructure struggling to cope.

The country spends 3.7% of its GDP on health care: a figure well below global average but on par with many of the countries around it. Although it has a network of multi-discipline hospitals, mainly in the more urban areas, doctors complain of low pay. Despite only being ranked at 187 on the World Health Organization's (WHO) league tables (World health report published in 2000) for the overall effectiveness of its health care system, a number of initiatives are improving life for inhabitants including family planning and immunisation programmes, and the country's prospects continue to change as its economy grows to become one of the largest in Africa.

South Africa

There is an excellent level of care to be found at the private hospitals in the major cities and around the game parks in South Africa, so much so, that it's not uncommon for patients to be flown in for treatment from other countries. This is against a backdrop of a poor standard of public health care and one of the shortest average life expectancies on the planet — it's fair to say that South Africa has more than its fair share of challenges.

As a whole, the country spends nearly 9% of its GDP on health care (on par with countries like Spain and Malta) but the doctor to population ratio is just under 1 to 1000, well below the world average. As public facilities can be poorly equipped, overcrowded, and waiting times long, comprehensive private medical insurance is worth thinking about for anyone looking to relocate to South Africa.

Kenya

With spending on health care just 5.7% of GDP, low by global standards, it is higher than that of some neighbouring countries like Sudan and Ethiopia. There is one doctor per 5,000 inhabitants and there can be huge variation in standards of care across geographical areas, private and public facilities, and the type of treatment available. The best private hospitals are to be found in the larger cities such as Nairobi and Mombasa, offering the kind of provision akin to that available in developed countries for many conditions.

Foreign nationals are able to join the national health insurance scheme (which is compulsory for civil service staff), but most have their own private insurance, often arranged through an employer. Consider having insurance in place to cover evacuation or repatriation, and set cash aside in case any payments need to be made up front.

Zimbabwe

Foreign nationals seeking to live and work in Zimbabwe might want to ensure they have adequate private medical insurance to cover private treatment and evacuation to somewhere with additional facilities, if necessary. The availability of staff, beds, technology, and pharmaceuticals is unreliable in hospitals and, although the government has promised to improve the health of the nation as a whole, many foreign nationals will find that provision is underfunded and varies in standard. Have access to enough cash to cover emergency care, as many private clinics will not treat patients until they have paid up front. With just 1 doctor per 10,000 people the country's health care system is ranked as 155th out of 191 in the world by the World Health Organization [22].

Zambia

Although Zambia has a basic public health care system, most newcomers and wealthier Zambians use the private system. With much of the international community and commerce based around Lusaka, this is where the best private hospitals are located. Those relocating to live in mining community compounds may find there are medical facilities on site, provided by their employer. The country as a whole spends 5% of its GDP on health care (less than a third of somewhere like the U.S.) and the health care system sits at position 182 out of 191 countries on WHO's league table. Public facilities are below the standard found in more developed countries and, with doctors receiving better pay in private hospitals and abroad, the country is struggling to keep its talent – there is roughly 1 doctor per 6,000 inhabitants (compared with nearly 5 for the same amount of people in South Africa).

Tanzania

One of the poorest countries in the world, the standard of health care facilities in Tanzania is low by global standards. There has been much improvement in recent years but challenges such as underfunding (just 5.6% of GDP, which translates as $51 per capita, compared to $4,000 per capita in the UK), chronic staff shortages (just one doctor per 30,000 inhabitants), and a lack of medical technology mean that provision is inadequate for both the population and foreign workers alike. Despite this, the health care system sits at 156th place on the WHO league table, which although poor is still above many neighbouring countries such as Mozambique and Zambia. The government does have a universal health care programme, but the quality and scarcity of facilities (generally only available in urban areas) mean that foreign nationals might want to think about having comprehensive private medical insurance, including cover for medical evacuation to other territories with higher standard facilities, such as Kenya and South Africa, in the event of a medical emergency.

Uganda

While the standard of medical facilities in Uganda is different to those found in developed countries, there are private clinics in Kampala that offer a good level of provision – some employing British doctors. Publicly run hospitals, and those in rural areas, may be overcrowded and under-stocked, and private clinics very expensive, so expats will want to consider having comprehensive private medical insurance. It's worth investigating whether the insurance covers treatment and evacuation to countries with better facilities, such as South Africa, as well as repatriation if necessary. English is commonly spoken across the country so a language barrier shouldn't be a problem. Uganda's health care system is ranked in <u>149th place out of 191 countries</u> in the world by WHO. There is roughly <u>one doctor per 1,000 people</u> (not dissimilar to many neighbouring states) and its population spends <u>7.2% of its GDP</u> on keeping healthy [22] .

NORDIC COUNTRIES:

The Nordic countries are Denmark, Finland, Iceland, Norway, and Sweden and comprise a total population of approximately 27 million. All five countries have welfare state models with universal and tax-funded health care systems, population-based nationwide registries, and personal identity numbers that enable individual level linkage of these registries.

People in the Nordic countries have universal access to the health care systems, which are mainly publicly financed through taxes with minor private health care sectors and limited private medical insurance. Approximately 2–10% of total in-hospital beds are private depending on the country. Moreover, private providers are often reimbursed by the public health insurance system according to economic contracts between the private and public sectors [23].

Population statistics for the five Nordic countries, 2018:

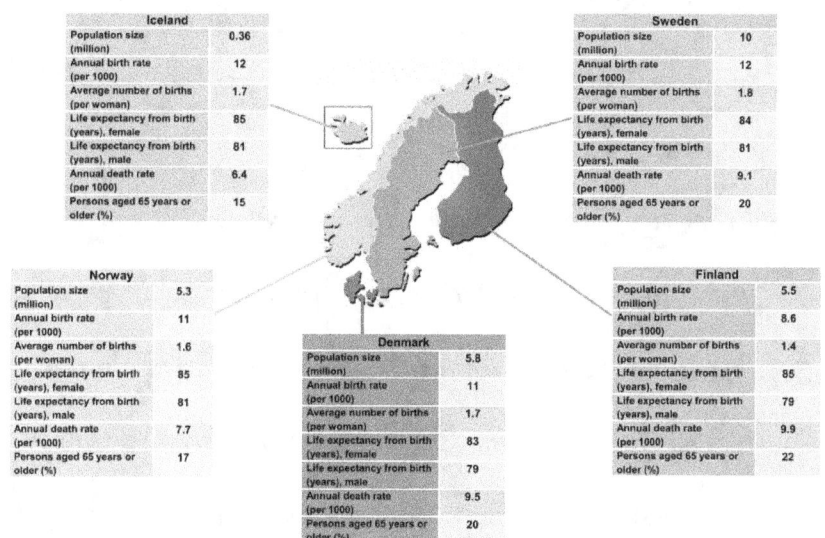

Overview of the operational organization of the Nordic health care systems:

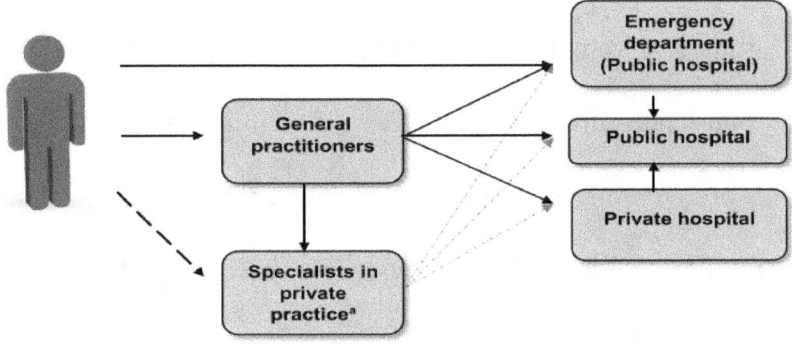

a Includes physiotherapists, dentists, psychologists, and specialized medical doctors working in private practice as eg. dermatologists, otorhinolaryngologist, fertility treatment specialists, cardiologists and pulmonologists. Visits to dentist never require referral from general practitioners (GPs). Other specialists may be accessed with or without referral from GPs; however, patient co-payment is often larger without a referral. Some private clinics are reimbursed completely or partly by public funding and some rely solely on patient self-payment or private insurance. Specialized medical doctors in private practice can refer patients to hospitals if needed. In Sweden, it is also possible to self-refer to hospital specialists. Patients need to fill out an online form, and then a hospital specialist will decide whether to see the patient without a GP referral.

THE DANISH HEALTH CARE SYSTEM:

Denmark is a country with approximately 5.8 million inhabitants and population statistics. In 2019, Denmark spent approximately 10% of its gross domestic product (GDP) on health care expenditures, corresponding to 5568 USD per capita Roughly 85% of all health care expenses are covered through taxes, including free access to general practitioners (GPs), hospitals, outpatient hospital specialist clinics, and partial reimbursement of prescribed medications. Patient co-payments are ~15% and primarily consist of cost-sharing for medications, physiotherapy, and/or dental care [23].

The Danish health care system is subdivided into primary and secondary health care sectors. Primary health care includes services provided by the regions, such as GPs and private clinics (dentists, psychologists, physiotherapists, chiropractors, and private practicing specialist), as well as services provided by the municipalities, such as elderly care, primary disease prevention, and rehabilitation. The secondary health care sector comprises hospitals, including inpatient treatment, outpatient hospital clinics, and emergency care, as well as psychiatric hospital care. GPs account for approximately 20% (n=4900) of the total Danish physician workforce and play a central role in the Danish health care system. GPs are generalists trained to evaluate the need for referral to specialists. Their primary tasks are to treat ordinary health problems, perform regular check-ups (eg, children and patients with chronic diseases), prescribe drugs and carry out vaccinations, refer patients to specialists when needed, and follow-up on patient health plans after hospital discharge. Except in emergencies, the GPs are the first point of contact and act as gatekeepers to the hospitals. GPs further provide on-call services after daily opening hours and on weekends for acute services. In case of emergencies, patients may go directly or by referral to public hospital emergency departments [24].

The Danish health care system currently has three administrative levels: the national level (state), the regional level (5 regions), and the local level (98 municipalities).

National Level (State):

The government, headed by The Ministry of Health, defines the framework of the Danish health care system by legislation, national guidelines, and health care monitoring. Furthermore, they set the economic framework and obtain financial agreements between the national, regional, and municipal administrative levels [24].

Regional Level:

The five regions are responsible for GPs, hospitals, specialists in private practice, and specialized nursing homes (eg, psychiatric patients). The regions also administer the Danish Drug Reimbursement Plan. In Denmark, all GPs are private practitioners but work according to a collective economic agreement and are paid by the public health insurance system with no patient cost-sharing (with few exceptions). Most specialists in private practice are also self-employed but are reimbursed for provided services on a fee-for-service basis according to an economic agreement with the regions.

Local Level (Municipalities):

The municipalities are responsible for social services and some health care services, including primary disease prevention and health promotion, student health, child dental care, ordinary home care and nursing homes, alcohol and drug abuse treatment, rehabilitation outside hospitals, and postnatal home visits [24].

THE SWEDISH HEALTH CARE SYSTEM:

Sweden is a country with approximately 10 million inhabitants and population statistics. The Swedish health care system is almost free of charge, with minor visit fees at GPs, outpatient hospital clinics, or during in-hospital stays. In 2019, Sweden spent 10.9% of their GDP on health care expenditures (5783 USD per capita). Tax incomes cover approximately 80% of the Swedish health care expenses, including services at GPs, hospitals, out-patient specialist clinics, and partial reimbursement of prescribed medications. Patient co-payments are ~20% and include visit fees, as well as co-payments for medications, physiotherapy, or dental care.

The operational organization of the Swedish health care system is subdivided into primary and secondary health care sectors. The primary health care sector includes GPs, psychologists, physiotherapists, some private practicing specialists, and rehabilitation. The secondary health care sector comprises hospitals, including inpatient and outpatient hospital clinic [25].

In Sweden, citizens are free to choose their primary care providers. The GPs can be the first point of contact, but citizens also have the opportunity to consult or self-refer to specialists through "1177.se", a 24-hour internet/phone health care service. A large proportion of Swedish patients have their initial health care contact with this service before seeking care with a physical health care provider. Through 1177.se, patients fill out an online or paper form and a specialist then decides whether to see the patient without contact with a GP first [26].

The Swedish health care system has three administrative levels: the national level (state), regional level (21 counties/regions), and local level (290 municipalities)

National Level (State):

The state, through the Ministry of Health and Social Affairs, outlines the Swedish health care system by legislation, guidelines, and health care monitoring [25].

Regional Level (Counties/Regions):

The Swedish counties/regions manage and operate the primary and secondary health care sectors. Primary care is provided by primary care units, approximately 42% of which are private but mostly still reimbursed by the public health insurance system. To work as a private practitioner within the social security system, an agreement (including economic agreement) must be made with the County Council. A number of private digital health care providers recently established themselves in Sweden. Their growth has been spurred, in part, by the COVID-19 pandemic [25, 27-28].

Local Level (Municipalities):

The Swedish municipalities are responsible for student health, nursing homes and home care, public health, disease prevention, and rehabilitation [25].

THE NORWEGIAN HEALTH CARE SYSTEM:

Norway is a country with approximately 5.3 million inhabitants and population statistics. The Norwegian health care system is universal with almost free access, though some patient fees exist when visiting GPs or outpatient hospital clinics. In 2019, Norway spent 10.5% of their GDP on health care expenditures (6647 USD per capita). Tax incomes cover approximately 85% of all health care expenses, including access to GPs, hospitals, outpatient hospital clinics, and partial reimbursement of prescribed medications. Patient co-payments are ~15% and are primarily co-payments for GP or outpatient clinic visits, and medications, or dental care.

The operational organization of the Norwegian health care system is divided into primary and secondary health care sectors. The primary health care sector includes GPs, psychologists, and physiotherapists among others. The secondary health care sector comprises hospitals, including inpatient care, outpatient hospital clinics, and psychiatric health care. GPs account for approximately 16% (n = 4900) of the total Norwegian physician workforce and have similar tasks as described for Denmark. As in the other Nordic countries, patients need a referral from their GP to access specialized care (e.g, hospital outpatient or inpatient care.

The Norwegian health care system is currently organized into three administrative levels: the national level (state), the regional level (4 regional health authorities), and the local level (356 municipalities). A few healthcare responsibilities (e.g, dental care) are held by the counties [29 - 30].

National Level (State):

The state (Ministry of Health and Care Services) determines the national health policy, decides on the allocation of funds within the health sector, and implements the national health policy. Furthermore, as the Ministry of Health and Care Services is the owner of the four regional health authorities, the ministry has somewhat direct responsibility for the delivery of hospital and specialist care.

Regional Level (Health Authorities):

The four regional health authorities (including 20 hospital trusts) are responsible for the hospitals and specialist out-patient hospital clinics, including psychiatric, rehabilitation and alcohol and substance abuse treatment.

Local Level (Municipalities) The Norwegian municipalities are responsible for social services and all primary health care, including GPs, rehabilitation, and physiotherapy, as well as public health and preventive measures. The majority of GPs are self-employed, but they are embedded in the public system through contracts with the municipalities, and patient cost-sharing is very limited [30].

THE FINNISH HEALTH CARE SYSTEM:

Finland is a country with approximately 5.5 million inhabitants and population statistics. The Finnish health care system is universal with almost free access, though some fees exist when visiting GPs, emergency rooms, outpatient clinics, or during inpatient hospital stays. In 2019, Finland spent 9.1% of their GDP on health care expenditures (4578 USD per capita). Taxes cover approximately 75% of all health care expenses, including access to GPs, hospitals, outpatient hospital clinics, and partial reimbursement of prescribed medications. Patient co-payments are ~20% and are primarily co-payments for visits and procedure fees, medication costs, or dental care. Private insurance covers approximately 5% of health care expenses [23].

The operational organization of the Finnish health care system is divided into primary, secondary, and tertiary healthcare. The primary health care sector includes GPs, dentists, psychologists, physiotherapists, some medical specialists, and rehabilitation. In addition, inpatient departments located in primary health centers are a specific feature of Finnish primary care. These inpatient hospitaltype wards are staffed with nurses, GPs, or specialists in geriatrics. The secondary health care sector includes regional hospitals (inpatient and outpatient specialist clinics). The tertiary sector includes university hospitals. GPs account for ~40% (n = 7000) of the total Finnish physician workforce and have similar tasks as described for Denmark. Patients need a referral from their GP to access the hospitals [31].

In 2019, the average number of visits to health care center per person was 4.1, of which 1.1 was a GP visit. A total of

67% of all Finns had used public primary health care in 2019 [23].

The Finnish health care system is currently structured into three administrative levels: the national level (state), the regional level (20 hospital districts), and the local level (311 municipalities) [31]. Finland has a decentralized health care system, meaning that responsibility for organizing, providing, and financing health care lies within the individual municipalities. A future task may be to implement a more centralized system [23].

National Level (State):

The state, headed by the Ministry of Social Affairs and Health, provides a framework for the Finnish health care system via health legislation.

Regional and Local Level (Municipalities):

The municipalities are responsible for organizing, providing, and financing primary care, as well as secondary and tertiary health care services through hospital districts. Due to the decentralized public administration, municipalities decide how the local services are provided, and differences may exist between the municipalities. Primary health care is provided at municipal health centers, where GPs are usually salaried employees of the municipalities. Yet, the lease of physicians from private firms has recently increased.13 The country is further divided into 20 hospital districts (plus Aland Islands, an autonomous area with special legislation) that are responsible for the provision of municipal secondary health care services. Hospital districts are federations of municipalities, and each municipality must be a member of a hospital district. Each hospital district is financed and managed by the member municipalities.

THE ICELANDIC HEALTH CARE SYSTEM:

Iceland is a country with approximately 0.36 million inhabitants and population statistics. People in Iceland have almost free access to the health care system with some minor fees for visits to GPs, out-patient hospital clinics and emergency wards [32]. In 2019, Iceland spent 8.8% of their GDP on health care expenditures (4811 USD per capita). Tax incomes cover approximately 80% of the Icelandic health care expenses, including services at GPs, hospitals, outpatient specialist clinics, and partial reimbursement of prescribed medications. Patient co-payments are ~20% and include visit fees and co-payments for medications, physiotherapy, or dental care [23].

The Icelandic health care system is divided into primary, secondary, and tertiary health care sectors. The primary health care sector includes GPs and primary health care clinics. The secondary sector includes private practicing specialists and the tertiary health care sector includes hospitals, comprising inpatient and outpatient hospital treatments, as well as psychiatric hospital care. From 1990–2017, Icelandic GPs had no gatekeeping role, but GP referrals have recently been re-implemented. GPs account for approximately 17% of the total Icelandic physician workforce. In 2019, approximately 80% of the population had contact with GPs (including visits and telephone consultancy) and 74% of the population actually visited a primary care center/ physician [33-35].

The Icelandic health care system is highly state-centralized and divided into a national level (state) and a regional level (7 regions). Local level administration plays a very minor role in the system.

National Level (State):

The state (the Ministry of Health) is responsible for health policy and the financing, planning, regulation, and delivery of both primary, secondary, and tertiary health care. The Ministry of Health acts through several agencies.

Physicians working in public hospitals and in general practice receive salaries from the state (with some fee-for-service payments to GPs for out of-hours work), as do other professionals (eg, nurses and midwives). Private practitioners, such as medical specialists who provide outpatient care outside of hospitals, physiotherapists, dentists, and psychologists are paid by the state on a fee-for-service basis.

Regional Level:

The country is divided into seven regions for healthcare organization purposes, but these regions have limited administrative authority [32].

4. HEALTH CARE DELIVERY IN SOUTHEAST ASIAN REGION

Singapore:

Private Health Insurance

Known as a medical centre of excellence in Southeast Asia, Singapore is home to a thriving health tourist industry. For elective, specialist surgery, and emergency treatment, medical insurance providers sometimes choose to evacuate their members to Singapore from other countries in the area. This excellent level of care does come at a price. The mandatory Medicare, and more comprehensive Medi shield insurance scheme, are open to those classed as permanent residents. This does not cover the majority of expatriates or almost any foreign workers, so they might want to consider private medical insurance.

The quality of care is supported by ten high-standard public hospitals, thirteen private and numerous other specialist clinics and treatment centres, in which English is commonly spoken. This is financed by 2.75% of the GDP and staffed by nearly 2 doctors per 1000 population. It's no wonder Singapore sits at number 6 of the World Health Organization (WHO) World health report, published in 2000 (based on health system attainment and performance in all member states, ranked by eight measures) [36].

Thailand

Thailand's health care system is delivered across private international and public government-funded hospitals. There's no access to free health care for non-nationals, so private medical insurance is worth investigating for expats in the country. Many public hospitals will ask for a guarantee of bill payment up front. This could mean providing the hospital with proof of preauthorisation (also known as Guarantee of Payment or Letter of Authorisation) from your health insurance provider. Private hospitals have excellent facilities, employing many English-speaking doctors, and usually have an International Liaison Department to help foreign nationals with medical insurance and financial matters.

The public system has limited nursing care, with the day-to-day well-being of patients being left to relatives. As a whole, the country is ranked at place 47 of the WHO league table for the performance of its health care. There are just 0.4 doctors per 1000 population with a shortage of general practitioners (GPs, also known as family doctors). The country spends 6.5% of its GDP on public health care (which is at the lower end of the world scale, comparable with countries like Cambodia and Indonesia).

Vietnam

Ranked at 160th place of 191 member states by the World Health Organization, the Vietnamese government has stepped up investment in its health care system in recent years and the country as a whole spends 7.1% of its GDP — more than many of its neighbours. There's a little over 1 doctor to 1,000 people — which is also a good ratio for this corner of Southeast Asia. In rural areas, standards are lower and you may be required to pay for treatment up front (even emergency care). But in the main cities such as Han Noi and Ho Chi Minh City, you can expect better facilities and English-speaking staff. Expats who don't speak English or Vietnamese might want to consider language support when accessing care or treatment. Before travelling to or relocating to Vietnam, it's could be worthwhile considering private medical insurance. There is no integrated care system (which means that there isn't an emergency ambulance service) and it's common for patients to be evacuated to Singapore or Thailand for certain conditions — so it's worth thinking about investing in appropriate medical insurance for these situations [36].

Malaysia

With a highly rated health care system across private and publicly funded hospitals, Malaysia's provision is ranked in 49th place on the WHO league table. Like most countries in the area, the best level of care is available in the larger cities and tourist areas. Recent increased investment in specialist doctors in areas such as cardiology and ophthalmology, has led to the country becoming a medical centre for excellence — with outsiders coming in for routine, emergency and elective procedures, such as plastic surgery.

The country spends 4.2% of the GDP on health care (comparable with India and Papua New Guinea), with a relatively low doctor ratio with 1 practitioner to 1,000 population. For foreign workers, a high level of care is available from good quality private and government hospitals, most with English-speaking doctors. Private medical insurance is mandatory (usually employer arranged) and it's important to note that you'll be required to provide a deposit before treatment, if you don't have adequate medical insurance cover.

Brunei Darussalam

A small but wealthy sultanate, Brunei Darussalam offers a good standard of health care which is free to citizens and permanent residents. The 40% of the population who are foreign nationals on work or tourist visas, however, need to pay for their health care. If you're relocating to, or visiting the country, you might want to investigate comprehensive private medical insurance. Apart from emergency treatment, hospitals will ask for a deposit or proof of cover before admitting a patient. The country has a major hospital in each of its four districts, the largest being in the capital Bandar Seri Begawan, and two excellent private facilities.

The wider health care system is rated as 20th in the world and is supported by a network of health clinics and a mobile flying service for more remote areas. There are no teaching hospitals, and because doctors are from overseas, foreign nationals are more likely to find a professional who speak English and other languages. There are 1.4 doctors per 1,000 population, a slightly higher ratio than neighbouring Malaysia [36].

Indonesia

Ranked in 92nd place by WHO and with only 1 doctor per 5000 population, Indonesia spends just 2.9% of its GDP on health care — one of the lowest rates in the world. The government has pledged investment and there is a fledgling universal health scheme but this is not open to expats. As many newcomers find themselves having to look further afield to Singapore and Australia for an adequate level of emergency care and elective treatment, private insurance is worth considering. Expats might also want to organise private ambulance cover, and private medical facilities are more likely to have staff who speak English as well as other languages.

Hong Kong

A wealthy, well-established commercial centre, everything in Hong Kong comes at a premium – including health care. Generally regarded as very expensive, there's a high standard of health care provision across both the public and private sectors. In public hospitals, which is better for things like general surgery and maternity care, there's a two-tier system of charging: 'eligible' rates and 'non-eligible' rates. The difference in cost between them is considerable and expats fall into the latter, more expensive category: non-eligible. Private hospitals also offer an excellent level of care. The island manufactures medical equipment, so it's no surprise medical facilities feature the latest technology across 12 internationally accredited private hospitals and 41 public ones. There's also an integrated system of clinics and smaller centres — all equally well equipped and monitored by the Department of Health. Comprehensive health care insurance is worth considering for foreign nationals — even considering the high costs — as the level of care received in return is of an excellent quality [36].

Note: Hong Kong is recognised as part of China by the WHO and so separate statistics for the territory are not provided in their reports.

5. HEALTH CARE DELIVERY IN INDIA

In 1920, the British government commissioned a report to suggest ways to structure their expanding health system investments. The commission chairman, Lord Bertrand Dawson, borrowing from previous experience in education, proposed three hierarchical levels of care locations (primary, secondary, tertiary). He and the commission first identified 'primary care' as the most basic level of a structured health system (akin to primary or elementary education), concerned with caring for simple, common problems in outpatient settings [37].

The concept of PHC has been repeatedly reinterpreted and redefined in the years since 1978, leading to confusion about the term and its practice. A clear and simple definition has been developed to facilitate the coordination of future PHC efforts at the global, national, and local levels and to guide their implementation: "PHC is a whole-of-society approach to health that aims at ensuring the highest possible level of health and well-being and their equitable distribution by focusing on people's needs and as early as possible along the continuum from health promotion and disease prevention to treatment, rehabilitation and palliative care, and as close as feasible to people's everyday environment." PHC entails three inter-related and synergistic components, including: comprehensive integrated health services that embrace primary care as well as public health goods and functions as central pieces; multi-sectoral policies and actions to address the upstream and wider determinants of health; and engaging and empowering individuals, families, and communities for increased social participation and enhanced self-care and self-reliance in health [38].

Health Administration System in India [5]:

At the state level

At the district level

Health Administration at the Centre:

Ministry of health and family welfare

Directorate general of health services

Central council of health and family welfare

Health Administration at the State Level:

State Ministry of Health

Ministry of Health & family welfare

Deputy ministry of Health & family welfare

State Health Directorate

Health Administration at the District Level Consists of six administrative areas:

1. Sub – divisions

2. Tehsils (Talukas)

3. Community development blocks

4. Municipalities & corporations

5. Villages

6. Panchayats

Health Care Systems in India:

In India it is represented by 5 major sectors which differ from each other by the Health technology applied and source of funds for the operation.

<u>(A) Public Health Sector</u>

a) Primary Health Care: Village level, Sub-centers, Primary health centers

b) Hospital/Health Centers: Community health centers, rural hospitals, District hospital/health center, Specialist hospitals, Teaching hospitals.

c) Health Insurance Schemes: Employee's state insurance scheme, Central government health scheme

d) Other Agencies: Defense services, Railways.

B) Private Sector: Private hospitals, Polyclinics, Nursing homes and dispensaries, General practitioners and clinics.

C) Indegenous Systems of Medicine: Ayurveda and Siddha, Unani and Tibbi, Homeopathy, Unregistered practitioners

D) Voluntary Health Agencies

E) National Health Programs: Primary Health Care in India: In 1977 the Rural Health Scheme launched [5].

INTEGRATED PRIMARY-SECONDARY CARE SYSTEM:

Health service integration is seen by the World Health Organization (WHO) as an essential requirement to achieve Universal Health Coverage (UHC). According to WHO, an integrated health service delivery is defined as: ... an approach to strengthen people-centred health systems through the promotion of the comprehensive delivery of quality services across the life-course, designed according to the multidimensional needs of the population and the individual and delivered by a coordinated multidisciplinary team of providers working across settings and levels of care, with feedback loops to continuously improve performance and to tackle upstream causes of ill health and to promote well-being through intersectoral and multisectoral action [39].

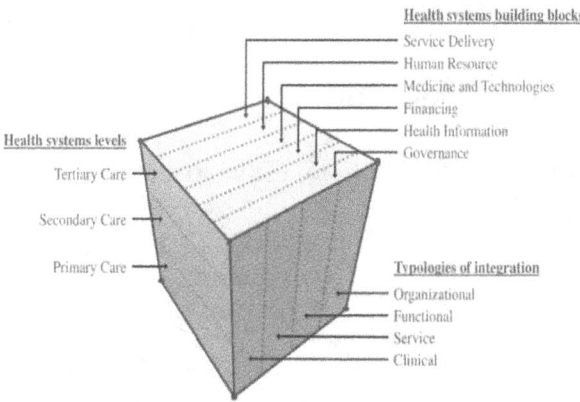

RURAL HEALTH CARE SYSTEM IN INDIA: [40]

Community health centre
Total no: 5649
Population coverage: 1 per 1,20,000 population in general areas and 1 per 80,000 population in difficult/tribal and hilly areas.

Primary health centre
Total no: 30,813
Population coverage: 1 per 30,000 population in general areas and 1 per 20,000 population in difficult/tribal and hilly areas

Sub Centres
Total no: 1,57,921
Population coverage: 1 per 5,000 population in general areas and 1 per 3,000 population in difficult/tribal and hilly areas

Indian Public Health System. Reprinted with permission from National Rural Health Mission, Ministry of Health and Family Welfare, Government of India [41]

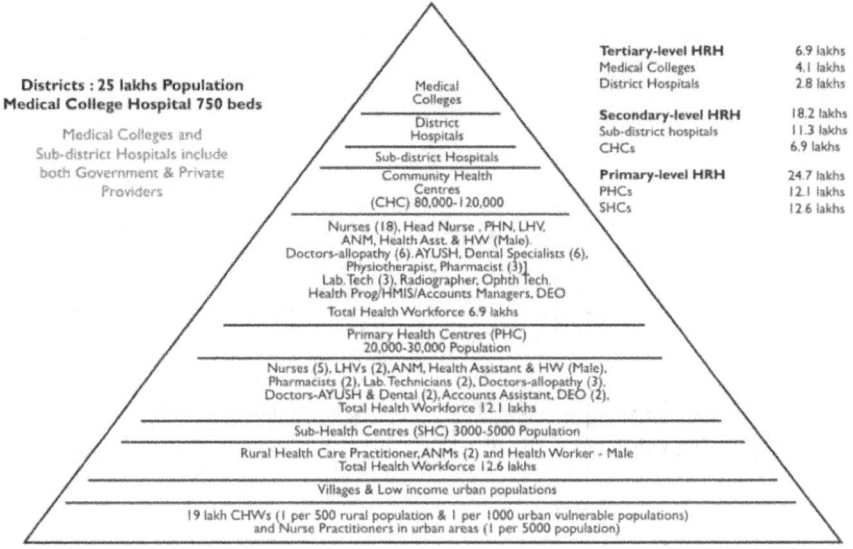

LEVELS OF HEALTH CARE SYSTEMS:

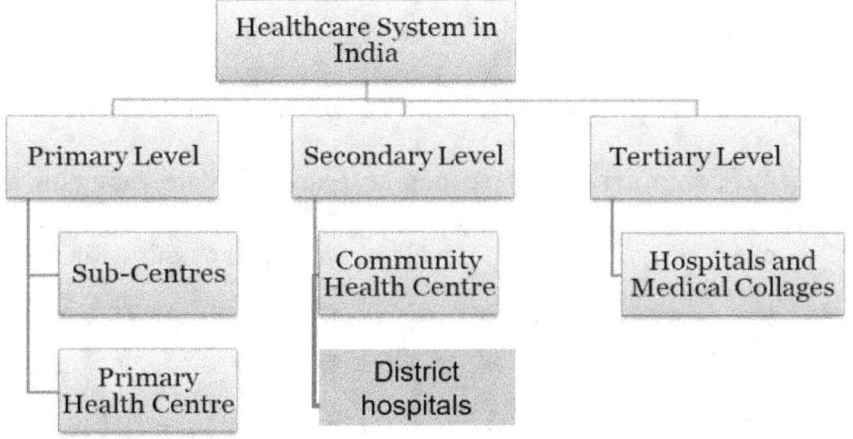

PRIMARY HEALTH CARE:

Alma-Ata conference (1978 by WHO and UNICEF) defined primary health care as follows: The approach has also been called as "health by the people" and "placing people's health in people's hands." Primary health care was accepted by the member countries of WHO as key to achieving the goal of "Health for All." Definition "Essential health care based on practical scientifically sound and socially acceptable methods and technology made universally accessible methods and technology made universally accessible to individuals and families in the community through their full participation and at a cost that the community and the country can afford to maintain at every stage of their development in the spirit of self-determination" [42].

Primary health care is based on principles of social justice, equity and right to health and in recognition of the fundamental right to the highest attainable standard of health, echoing Article 25 of the Universal Declaration on Human Rights. It is an integral part of overall social and economic development in addition to catering to the healthcare needs of the country. Health and Wellness Centre – Sub Health Centre / Urban Health and Wellness Centre (HWC-SHCs/ UHWCs) strive to provide affordable, accessible, practical, quality and socially acceptable healthcare to the community and is universally available, regardless of their economic stature or payment capacity. Primary healthcare services in India are currently being delivered through Sub-Centres and Primary Health Centres in rural areas and Urban Primary Health Centres in urban areas.

PRINCIPAL OF PRIMARY HEALTH CARE:

1. Equitable distribution

Health services must be shared equally by all people irrespective of their ability to pay, and all (rich or poor, urban or rural) must have access to health services. At present, health services are mainly concentrated in the major towns and cities resulting in inequality of care to the people in rural areas. The worst hit are the needy and vulnerable groups of the population in rural areas and urban slums. This has been termed as social injustice. Primary health care aims to redress this imbalance by shifting the centre of gravity of the health care system from cities (where three-quarters of the health budget is spent) to the rural areas (where three-quarters of the people live), and bring these services as near people's homes as possible [5].

2. Community participation

Notwithstanding the overall responsibility of the Central and State Governments, the involvement of individuals, families, and communities in promotion of their own health and welfare, is an essential ingredient of primary health care. There must be a continuing effort to secure meaningful involvement of the community in the planning, implementation and maintenance of health services, besides maximum reliance on local resources such as manpower, money and materials. In short, primary health care must be built on the principle of community participation (or involvement). One approach that has been tried successfully in India is the use of village health guides and trained dais. They are selected by the local community and trained locally in the delivery of primary health care to the community they belong, free of charge. By overcoming cultural and communication barriers, they provide primary health care in ways that are acceptable to the community. It is now considered that "health guides" and trained dais are an essential feature of primary health care in India. These concepts are revolutionary.

3. Intersectoral coordination

There is an increasing realization of the fact that the components of primary health care cannot be provided by the health sector alone. The Declaration of Alma-Ata states that "primary health care involves in addition to the health sector, all related sectors and aspects of national and community development, in particular agriculture, animal husbandry, food, industry, education, housing, public works, communication and others sectors". To achieve such cooperation, countries may have to review their administrative system, reallocate their resources and introduce suitable legislation to ensure that coordination can take place. This requires strong political will to translate values into action. An important element of intersectoral approach is planning - planning with other sectors to avoid unnecessary duplication of activities.

4. Appropriate technology

Appropriate technology has been defined as "technology that is scientifically sound, adaptable to local needs, and acceptable to those who apply it and those for whom it is used, and that can be maintained by the people themselves in keeping with the principle of self-reliance with the resources the community and country can afford". The term "appropriate" is emphasized because in some countries, large, luxurious hospitals that are totally inappropriate to the local needs, are built, which absorb a major part of the national health budget, effectively blocking any improvement in general health services. This also applies to using costly equipment, procedures and techniques when cheaper, scientifically valid and acceptable ones are available, viz, oral rehydration fluid, standpipes which are socially acceptable, and financially more feasible than house-to-house connections, etc. It will be seen from the above discussion that primary care is qualitatively a different approach to deal with the health problems of a community. Unlike the previous approaches (e.g, basic health services, integrated health care, vertical health services) which depended upon taking health services to the doors of the people, primary health care approach starts with the people themselves. This approach signifies a new dynamism in health care and has been described as Health by the people, placing people's health in people's hands. The ends of the primary health care approach are the same as those of earlier approaches (i.e., attainment of an acceptable level of health by every individual), but the means adopted are different, that is, more equitable distribution and nation-wide coverage, more intersectoral coordination and more community involvement in health-related matters. In short, primary health care goes beyond the conventional health services. It forms part of the larger concept of Human Resources and Development [5].

ELEMENTS OF PRIMARY HEALTH CARE:

Although specific services provided will vary in different countries and communities, the Alma-Ata Declaration has outlined 8 essential components of primary health care.

1. Education concerning prevailing health problems and the methods of preventing and controlling them;

2. Promotion of food supply and proper nutrition;

3. An adequate supply of safe water and basic sanitation;

4. Maternal and child health care, including family planning;

5. Immunization against major infectious diseases;

6. Prevention and control of locally endemic diseases;

7. Appropriate treatment of common diseases and injuries;

8. Provision of essential drugs [5].

PRIMARY HEALTH CENTRES AND SUB-CENTRES;

Primary level health care in India:

India has a rich past in the field of medical sciences. Both physical and mental health were considered important parameters of health. The 'Charaka Samhita" was the mainstay for medicine for centuries and "Sushruta Samhita" was the ancient medical compendium of surgery compiled around 6th century B.C. The Buddhist era in the 6th century B.C. saw the establishment of "Viharas" - monasteries for the care of the sick, impoverished, and disabled, as well as medical education. Several hospitals were operational throughout King Ashoka's reign in the 2nd century B.C. Modern hospitals and healthcare systems were constructed. From the late 19th century through the early 20th century, the first medical colleges were established for organized medical training. Further, dispensaries were established at sub-division and district level and hospitals at provincial level were attached to medical colleges. The present focus of public health evolved slowly across the globe. The broad foundations of public health later evolved when Winslow defined public health as "the science and art of preventing disease, prolonging life, and promoting health through the organized efforts and informed choices of society, organizations, public and private communities, and individuals." [43].

The Alma Ata Declaration:

The International Conference on Primary Health Care held in Alma-Ata in 1978 remains at the heart of discussions on public health, health policy, and human development [44]. The 134 member states of the WHO declared good health was also the result of factors that included access to services, education, social and economic status and political and individual choices. The Alma Ata Declaration stated 'Governments have a responsibility for the health of their people which can be fulfilled only by the provision of adequate health and social measures. The people have the right and duty to participate individually and collectively in the planning and implementation of their health care'. The Declaration supported by all member states of WHO put forward a new policy titled Primary Health Care (PHC) defined as 'essential health care based on practical, scientifically sound and socially acceptable methods and technology made universally accessible to individuals and families in the community through their full participation and at a cost that the community country can afford to maintain at every stage of their development in the spirit of self-reliance and self- determination'[45].

The International Conference on Primary Health Care, meeting in Alma-Ata this twelfth day of September in the year Nineteen hundred and seventy-eight, expressing the need for urgent action by all governments, all health and development workers, and the world community to protect and promote the health of all the people of the world [46].

<u>Primary health care:</u>

1. Reflects and evolves from the economic conditions and sociocultural and political characteristics of the country and its communities and is based on the application of the relevant results of social, biomedical and health services research and public health experience;

2. Addresses the main health problems in the community, providing promotive, preventive, curative and rehabilitative services accordingly;

3. Includes at least: education concerning prevailing health problems and the methods of preventing and controlling them; promotion of food supply and proper nutrition; an adequate supply of safe water and basic sanitation; maternal and child health care, including family planning;

immunization against the major infectious diseases; prevention and control of locally endemic diseases; appropriate treatment of common diseases and injuries; and provision of essential drugs;

4. Involves, in addition to the health sector, all related sectors and aspects of national and community development, in particular agriculture, animal husbandry, food, industry, education, housing, public works, communications and other sectors; and demands the coordinated efforts of all those sectors;

5. Requires and promotes maximum community and individual self-reliance and participation in the planning, organization, operation and control of primary health care, making fullest use of local, national and other available resources; and to this end develops through appropriate education the ability of communities to participate;

6. Should be sustained by integrated, functional and mutually supportive referral systems, leading to the progressive improvement of comprehensive health care for all, and giving priority to those most in need;

7. Relies, at local and referral levels, on health workers, including physicians, nurses, midwives, auxiliaries and community workers as applicable, as well as traditional practitioners as needed, suitably trained socially and technically to work as a health team and to respond to the expressed health needs of the community [46].

PRIMARY HEALTH CENTRES (PHC)

The primary health care system in India has evolved since independence and there is an elaborate network of nearly 200,000 Government Primary Health Care Facilities

(GPHCFs), both in rural and urban areas. The existing GPHCFs deliver a narrow range of services, due to variety of reasons including, at times, the non-availability of providers as well. Thus, the GPHCFs in India are grossly underutilized & excluding for the mother and child health services, in 2013-14, only 11.5% of rural and 3.9% in urban people in need of health services used this vast network. People in India either choose higher level of government facilities for primary health care (PHC) needs (which results in an issue of subsidiarity) or attend a private provider (which results in the out-of-pocket expenditure or OOPE), both situations are not good for a well-functioning health system. The challenge of weak PHC in India are increasingly being recognized and acknowledged. The National Health Policy (NHP) 2017 of India proposed to strengthen PHC systems, invest two-third or more government health spending on PHC, with an increase in overall government funding for health to 2.5% of Gross

Domestic Product (GDP) by 2025, against 1.18% in 2015–16. Following on the NHP 2017, the Government in India announced Ayushman Bharat Program (ABP) in February 2018 with two components of (a) Health and Wellness Centres (HWCs) to strengthen & deliver comprehensive Primary Health Care (cPHC) services for entire population and (b) Pradhan Mantri Jan Arogya Yojana (PMJAY) for secondary and tertiary level hospitalization services for bottom 40% of families in India [47]

Primary Health Centres essentially deliver preventive, promotive, basic curative, palliative, and rehabilitative services encompassing community and programmatic requirements. Primary healthcare services in India have till now been delivered through Sub-centres and Primary Health Centres in rural areas and Urban Primary Health Centres in urban areas. In February 2018, the Government of India announced 1,50,000 Ayushman Bharat- Health and Wellness Centres (AB-HWCs) to be established across the country by December 2022. The existing Sub- Health Centres (SHC), Primary Health Centres (PHC) and Urban Primary Health Centres (UPHC) are being transformed into AB-HWCs to deliver Comprehensive Primary Health Care (CPHC) that includes preventive, promotive, curative, palliative and rehabilitative services which are universal, free, and closer to the community. Since the last revision of the IPHS in 2012, a number of new initiatives, interventions, programmes and projects have been introduced in the public health system.

The National Health Policy, 2017 recommended strengthening the delivery of Primary Health Care, through establishment of "Health and Wellness Centres", as the platform to deliver Comprehensive Primary Health Care with the principle of "time to care" to be no more than 30 minutes. To accommodate these developments, it is essential to incorporate them in existing IPHS so that the revised IPHS 2022 are informed by stakeholder feedback about the relevance and usefulness of these standards and remain fit-for-purpose in light of emerging evidence and advancements in health, science, and technology [43]

The broad objectives of the Indian Public Health Standards (IPHS) for PHC in rural and urban areas include the following:

1. To define uniform benchmark to ensure high quality services that are accountable, responsive, and sensitive to the needs of the community.

2. To specify the minimum assured (essential) and achievable (desirable) services that are expected to be provided at different levels of public health facilities.

3. To provide guidance on health systems strengthening components which includes architectural design of facilities, human resources for health, drugs, diagnostics,

equipment, administrative and logistical support services to improve the overall health related outcomes

4. To achieve and maintain an acceptable standard of the quality of care at public facilities

5. To facilitate monitoring and supervision of the facilities

6. To provide guidance and tools for governance, leadership and evaluation.

Revised IPHS 2022 guidelines classify the rural and urban PHC as:

		Population norm for HWC-PHC	
S. No.	Type of PHC facility	Plain (population)	Hilly and Tribal areas (population)
1	Rural PHC	30,000	20,000
2	Urban PHC	50,000	--
3	Polyclinic	2.5 lakh - 3 lakh	--

a) HWC-PHCs:

Ideally, for rural areas, the states should aspire to make all PHCs functional as 24x7 facilities. However, there is a need to prioritize PHCs conducting deliveries to function as 24x7 HWC-PHCs. All other PHCs should continue to provide routine care along with preventive and promotive health interventions and function as PHCs-HWCs.

b) Urban HWC-PHCs:

In urban areas, assured round-the-clock emergency and secondary care services are readily available, so primary health centres are expected to provide routine OPD care along with preventive and promotive health interventions and function as UPHCs-HWCs. However, the UPHCs with indoor beds already conducting deliveries can continue to function as 24x7 UPHCs-HWCs.

c) Specialist UPHC/Polyclinic (Urban):

"Multispecialty UPHC/Polyclinics" in urban areas should be established with the aim to further reduce morbidity and mortality by providing specialist services on ambulatory/day care basis, closer to the urban community. Such poly clinic services would be limited to outpatient care [43].

Service Provision:

Presently even a well-functioning primary health centre provides services that are limited to reproductive, sexual and child health along with some of the National Disease Control Programmes. Together these conditions, for which people seek health care, represent less than 15% of all services. For all the rest, people have no option but to resort to either the local private care provider or travel to the crowded District Hospital or Medical College hospital.

Ayushman Bharat with its two inter-related components of Health and Wellness Centres (HWCs) and the Pradhan Mantri Jan Arogya Yojana (PM-JAY) represents a paradigm shift towards India's path to Universal Health

Coverage (UHC). While PM-JAY is the largest health assurance scheme in the world which caters to BPL and certain other categories of the Indian population for secondary and tertiary care hospitalization, the AB- HWCs are envisaged to deliver an expanded range of comprehensive primary healthcare services which address the basic primary healthcare needs of the entire population in their area. The two combined, expand access, universality, and equity in health care service delivery in the country.

Primary healthcare plays a major role in delivering comprehensive set of services. In addition to the basic curative services of primary care level, Health and Wellness Centres have an important role in the prevention of several disease conditions, including both communicable and non-communicable diseases. They are envisaged to deliver people centred, holistic, equity sensitive response to people's health needs through a process of population enumeration, facility based and outreach services, regular home-based and community interactions and improve people's participation. A community based participatory approach, which ensures preventive and promotive actions, considered as a priority for health, is the primary objective of these centres.

The twelve packages envisaged under Comprehensive Primary Healthcare services (CPHC) are:

1. Care in Pregnancy and Childbirth

2. Neonatal and Infant Health Care Services

3. Childhood and Adolescent Health Care Services

4. Family Planning, Contraceptive Services, and other Reproductive Health Care Services

5. Management of Communicable Diseases: National Health Programmes

6. General Out-patient Care for Acute Simple Illnesses and Minor Ailments

7. Screening, Prevention, Control and Management of Non-communicable Diseases

8. Care for Common Ophthalmic and ENT Problems

9. Basic Oral Health Care

10. Elderly and Palliative Health Care Services

11. Emergency Medical Services including Burns and Trauma

12. Screening and Basic Management of Mental Health Ailments

<u>Jan Arogya Samiti:</u>

The Jan Arogya Samiti serve as institutional platform of SHC/UHWC and PHC/UPHC level AB-HWCs in both rural and urban areas, for community participation in its management, governance and ensuring accountability, with respect to provision of healthcare services and amenities. They support AB-HWC team in working with VHSNCs/MAS, and serve as an umbrella, providing mentorship for Health Promotion and Action on Social and Environmental Determinants of Health, in community level activities of National Health Programmes and other community interventions. JAS also support and facilitate the conduct of activities pertaining to social accountability at AB-HWC in coordination with VHSNCs/MAS and act as Grievance Redressal Platform for families who access healthcare services at AB- HWCs, ensuring availability and accountability for quality services. JAS facilitate and support Gram Panchayats/Urban Local Bodies (ULBs) of the area in undertaking health planning. At the facility level, the JAS members will identify gaps related to physical infrastructure, services (essential and desirable), human resources (HR), equipment, drugs, and diagnostics at PHC level based on the standards prescribed here [43].

Minimum Performance Standards for human resource for health in PHC:

S. No.	Staff	Break up of activities
1	General Medicine	• OPD = 60 pts/day • Invasive Procedures= 10 Procedures/week
2	Obstetrics & Gynecologist	• OPD= 60 pts/day
3	Pediatrician	• OPD= 60 pts/day • Invasive Procedures= 10 Procedures/week
4	Ophthalmologist	• OPD= 60 pts/day • OT= 7 major surgeries/week
5	Dermatologist	• OPD= 60 patient/day • Minor Procedures (Skin biopsies, cauterization etc.) 10 Procedures/week
6	Psychiatrist	• OPD= 20-30 pts/day • Consultation for referred patient
7	Medical Officer	• OPD = 75 patient/day • IPD 10 pts per/Day • OT assistance, emergency and other duties
8	Dentist	• OPD = 20 pts/day • Dental Procedures= 8-10 (30 min./patient)
9	Staff nurse	As per INC norms (for OPD, IPD shifts and specialist services)
10	Medical Laboratory Technologist/Lab Technician	100 tests/day (semi-autoanalyzer), 200 tests/day (autoanalyzer)
11	Physiotherapist	15-20 physiotherapy intervention/day (15-20 minutes/service) Physiotherapy advice for IPD patient
12	Counsellor	20-25 counselling sessions (Group/Interpersonal)/day (10-15 min/patient for interpersonal counselling)
13	Optometrist/Ophthalmic Assistant/Vision Technician	• 30-40 cases per day. • 10-12 min/pts for refractive assessment • Detection of cataract and other basic EYE ailments • Appropriate referrals • Linkages with RBSK team for refraction and issue of spectacles.
14	Dental Assistant	• Assist the Dentist during dental procedures • Maintain dental laboratory records. • Ensuring adherence to infection prevention protocols including sterilization.
15	Pharmacist	120 dispensations of prescription/day, maintain stock registers, store, inventory management

All "Minimum Assured Services" or Essential Services as envisaged in the PHC should be available. The services which are indicated as Desirable are for the purpose that we should aspire to achieve for this level of facility. Appropriate guidelines for each National Programme for management of routine and emergency cases are being provided to the PHC [43].

HEALTH AND WELLNESS CENTRES – SUB HEALTH CENTRES / URBAN HEALTH AND WELLNESS CENTRES:

HWC-SHCs/UHWCs strive to provide affordable, accessible, practical, quality and socially acceptable healthcare to the community and is universally available, regardless of their economic stature or payment capacity. Primary healthcare services in India are currently being delivered through Sub-Centres and Primary Health Centres in rural areas and Urban Primary Health Centres in urban areas.

To meet all these national and international commitments, it is essential for public health facilities to deliver quality services through defined standards known as the Indian Public Health Standards (IPHS). It provides guidance on the health system components such as infrastructure, human resource, drugs, diagnostics, equipment, quality and governance requirements for delivering health services at these facilities.

In the year 2005, National Rural Health Mission (now National Health Mission) was launched for "attainment of universal access to equitable, affordable and quality health care services, accountable & responsive to people's needs, with effective inter-sectoral convergent action to address the wider social determinants of health". Also, recently the Astana Declaration in October 2018 endorsed emphasizing the critical role of primary health care around the world.

The declaration aims to refocus efforts on primary health care to ensure that everyone everywhere is able to enjoy the highest possible attainable standard of health. To address the morbidity burden and the social determinants, increased community participation, surveillance, health promotion, engaging with information technologies (IT) and for ensuring continuum of care; the Government of India implemented the holistic programme "Ayushman Bharat", which comprises of two inter-related components. The first component involves upgradation of all the Sub Health Centres (SHCs), Primary Health Centres (PHCs) and Urban Primary Health Care Centres (UPHCs) to Health and Wellness Centres (HWCs) for the delivery of comprehensive primary health care. The second component comprises of Ayushman Bharat Pradhan Mantri Jan Arogya Yojana (PMJAY) which aims to provide financial protection for secondary and tertiary care to socially vulnerable and low-income households. Thus, together, the two components of Ayushman Bharat will enable the country to achieve Universal Health Coverage and eventually "Health for All".

The HWCs will provide an expanded range of services beyond the selective package of health care for pregnant women, children, reproductive health and communicable diseases. These HWCs will also deliver Preventive, Promotive, Curative, Rehabilitative and Palliative care services close to communities with the principle being 'time to care' to be not more than 30 minutes from the farthest village. The HWCs are envisaged to provide clinical management for most common ailments, prompt referral to doctor or for specialist consultations at higher facilities and undertake follow-up of down referrals. For effective and quality delivery of comprehensive healthcare services, it is essential for public health facilities to adopt uniform standards and norms. The defined uniform standards had been envisaged to deliver quality services to citizens with dignity and respect and provide guidance on the health system components such as infrastructure, human resource, drugs, diagnostics, equipment, quality and governance requirements for delivering seamless health services at these public facilities [48].

The broad objectives of the Indian Public Health Standards (IPHS) for HWC-SHC and UHWCs include the following:

1. To define uniform benchmark to ensure high quality services that are accountable, responsive, and sensitive to the needs of the community.

2. To specify the minimum assured (essential) and achievable (desirable) services that are expected to be provided at different levels of public health facilities.

3. To provide guidance on health systems strengthening components which includes architectural design of facilities, human resources for health, drugs, diagnostics,

equipment, administrative and logistical support services to improve the overall health related outcomes

4. To achieve and maintain an acceptable standard of quality of care at public health facilities

5. To facilitate monitoring and supervision of the facilities

6. To provide guidance and tools for governance, leadership and evaluation.

<u>Revised IPHS 2022 guidelines classify the HWCs – SHC/ UHWC as:</u>

1. Health and Wellness Centres - Primary Health Centre:

   a) HWC-PHC in rural areas
   b) HWC- UPHC in urban areas

2. Health and Wellness Centres - Sub Health Centre:

   a) Health and Wellness Centre - Sub Health Centre in rural areas
   b) Urban Health & Wellness Centre in urban areas

S. No.	Type of PHC facility	Population norm for HWC-SHC/UHWC	
		Plain (population)	Hilly/Tribal (population)
1	HWC-SHC	5000	3000
2	UHWC	15,000- 20,000	-

Health and Wellness Centres have an important role in the prevention of several disease conditions, including non-communicable diseases and health promotion. They go beyond first contact care and mediate an assured two-way referral service to primary and secondary level facilities. They also play an important role in undertaking public health functions in the community leveraging the frontline workers and community platforms. They are envisaged to deliver people Centred, holistic, equity sensitive, quality response to people's health needs through a process of population enumeration, regular home and community interactions and improving people's participation. A community based participatory approach which ensures preventive and promotive actions for health is considered as one of the primary objectives of these Centres. The healthcare services to be provided at these Centres include health promotion, early identification, ensuring treatment adherence, follow-up care, ensuring continuity of care by appropriate referrals, optimal home and community follow-up, disease surveillance, and health promotion and prevention for the expanded range of CPHC services [49].

The twelve packages envisaged under Comprehensive Primary Healthcare services (CPHC) are same as HWC – SHC.

In addition to providing clinical services, HWCs are also to be utilized as a platform for teleconsultation and expanding the range of diagnostics. As defined in this guideline states can add more tests in hub & spoke model with a nearest CHC/UCHC if range of diagnostics is to be expanded particularly in urban areas. To ensure continuum of care, assured referral with facility readiness to manage referred cases must be established with the PHC/UPHC and secondary level facilities in rural and urban areas. The referral transport network should have the requisite number of equipped ambulances (depending on population norms) and adequately trained human resources.

Apart from other services, an integration of Yoga and AYUSH services as appropriate to people's needs are required for provision of all-inclusive health services. The emphasis on health promotion (including the School Health and Wellness Ambassador Initiative) for public health action through active engagement and capacity building of community platforms, elected representatives and community volunteers is envisioned.

Besides facility-based services, HWCs play an important role in community outreach, which will be a part of the service package at HWCs (e.g., VHNDs/UHNDs). Need based outreach sessions can be conducted without any fixed periodicity (at required intervals), depending on national program requirements and for inter-departmental convergence activities from time-to-time basis in any particular area. Program specific outreach camps for screening and early detection of diseases such as TB, leprosy, fever, hypertension, diabetes, asthma, glaucoma, blindness, etc., special health drives, vaccination drives, health camps for disease specific awareness generation or other program related activities, convergence activities with other departments for health promotion/awareness generation by addressing social determinants of health such as sanitation, water, gender issues, violence, substance abuse, etc., public health surveillance, outbreak investigation in case of any outbreaks, epidemics and pandemics, Disaster mitigation/ disaster management activities in case of floods, droughts, earthquakes, landslides, etc., targeted interventions for migrants population sub groups residing in urban areas are some of the examples of such outreach sessions.

All infrastructure plans and human resource requirements should be based on the range of services to be provided at that facility. The services to be provided at both types of facilities are identified as 'essential' and 'desirable'. The former includes those 'minimum assured services' that every facility at that level must provide. Desirable services are those that a facility should aspire to ultimately achieve (if not already being provided) over a period of time depending on the needs of community [49].

Minimum assured services HWC-SHC:

S. No.	Human Resource required	Required Numbers
1.	Community Health Officer (CHO)	1
2.	Multipurpose Health Worker	1 Male +1 Female

Sanitation and security services can be hired/outsourced

There should be one ASHA per 1000 population or one ASHA per habitation in tribal, hilly and desert areas should be attached with the HWC as part of the entire team

Minimum assured services UHWC:

S. No.	Human Resource	Required Numbers
1.	Medical Officer	1
2.	Staff Nurse	1
3.	MPW (Male)	1
4.	Sanitary Staff *	1
5.	Security Staff**	1

*Sanitation and security services** can be hired/outsourced

One ASHA per 2000 population and one ANM per 10000 population should be attached as part of the entire team in urban areas. IPHS 2022 has not calculated leave reserves for any level of staff. However, states have the flexibility to determine their own level of 'leave reserve' to be sanctioned and this additional number of nurses and allied health professionals can be deployed to cover for leave and absences. Leave and Training Reserves of 15% or as per the state rule is recommended for all staff in IPHS.

Minimum Performance Standards (HR):

S. No.	Staff	Break up of activities
1.	Medical officer	OPD = 75 patient /day
		Clinical, Emergency and other duties
		Supervision of Public Health and health programmes related activities.
2.	CHO	OPD = 20 patient /day
		Tele consultations= 40-50 per month
		Clinical, Emergency and other duties
		Supervision of Public Health and health programmes related activities.
3.	Staff nurse	As per INC norms (for OPD, IPD shifts and specialist services)
4.	Pharmacist	120 dispensations of prescription/day, maintain stock registers, store, inventory management

Note: Assuming 8 hours shift and 75% productivity and efficiency, it is estimated that there will be 6 hours of working time spread over 6 days in a week

ACCREDITED SOCIAL HEALTH ACTIVIST (ASHA):

The Anganwadi (AW)—meaning courtyard, is a childcare centre located within the village or the slum area itself. It is the centre point for the delivery of services at community levels to children below six years of age, adolescent girl's pregnant women, and nursing mothers. The AW is a meeting ground where groups of women/mothers can come together, with other frontline workers, to promote awareness and joint action for child development and women's empowerment. All services of the Integrated Child Development Services (ICDS) are provided through the AW in an integrated manner to enhance their impact on childcare. Each AW is run by an Anganwadi worker (AWW) supported by a helper in integrated service delivery, and improved linkages with the health system— thus increasing the capacity of community and women, especially mothers for childcare, development and survival. They provide services like, pre-school formal education, nutrition and health education supplementary nutrition, referral services, Auxiliary Nurse Midwife (ANM) in immunization, health check-ups. AWWs are trained regularly on Behaviour Change Communication (BCC) and capacity building strategies along with health education [49].

ASHA will be the first port of call for any health-related demands of deprived sections of the population, especially women and children, who find it difficult to access health services [50].

The details task assigned to ASHA workers under National Health Mission:

1. To create awareness and provide information to the community on determinants of health such as nutrition, basic sanitation and hygienic practices, healthy living and working conditions, information on existing health services and the need for timely use of health services.

2. To counsel women and families on birth preparedness, importance of safe delivery, breastfeeding and complementary feeding, immunization, contraception and prevention of common infections including Reproductive Tract Infection/Sexually Transmitted Infection (RTIs/STIs) and care of the young child.

3. To mobilize the community and facilitate people's access to health and health related services available at the village/sub-centre/primary health centres, such as Immunization, Ante Natal Check-up (ANC), Post Natal Check-up (PNC), ICDS, sanitation and other services being provided by the government.

4. To work with the Village Health, Sanitation and Nutrition Committee to develop a comprehensive village health plan, and promote convergent action by the committee on social determinants of health. In support with VHSNC, ASHAs will assist and mobilize the community for action against gender-based violence.

5. To arrange escort/accompany pregnant women & children requiring treatment/ admission to the nearest pre- identified health facility i.e., Primary Health Centre/Community Health Centre/First Referral Unit (PHC/CHC/FRU).

6. To provide community level curative care for minor ailments such as diarrhoea, fevers, care for the normal and sick new-born, childhood illnesses and first aid. She will be a provider of Directly Observed Treatment Short-course (DOTS) under Revised National Tuberculosis Control Programme. She will also act as a depot holder for essential health products appropriate to local community needs. A Drug Kit will be provided to each ASHA. Contents of the kit will be based on the recommendations of the expert/technical advisory group set up by the Government of India. These will be updated from time to time, States can add to the list as appropriate.

7. To act as a care provider can be enhanced based on state needs. States can explore the possibility of graded training to the ASHA to provide palliative care, screening for non-communicable diseases,

childhood disability, mental health, geriatric care and others.

8. To provide information on about the births and deaths in her village and any unusual health problems/disease outbreaks in the community to the Sub-Centres/Primary Health Centre. She will promote construction of household toilets under Total Sanitation Campaign [51].

<u>Anganwadi Workers (AWWs):</u>

(i) Growth monitoring: The growth measurement Length/Height & weight is essential for all children to obtain their status as Normal, Underweight, Severe Acute Malnutrition (SAM), Moderate Acute Malnutrition (MAM), Stunted and Wasted. The measurement should be done for at least 80% of children in 0-6 age group every month. Any child which is not measured in a particular month has to be compulsorily measured next month.

(ii) Home visits: Completing at least 60 percent of home visits to pregnant women, lactating mothers and children up to two years of age as per the home visit scheduler.

Anganwadi Helpers (AWHs): Opening the Anganwadi Centre (AWC): Opening the AWC for at least 21 days in the month [52].

SECONDARY HEALTHCARE:

Secondary Healthcare refers to a second tier of health system, in which patients from primary health care are referred to specialists in higher hospitals for treatment. In India, the health centres for secondary health care include

District hospitals and Community Health Centre at block level [53].

The delivery of services through the public health sector in India follows the three-tier structure of primary, secondary, and tertiary health care services. This covers both rural and urban areas. While health services in rural areas have always been an integral part of the public health sector, focus on urban health came during Reproductive and Child Health (RCH) – I and continued in RCH-II as part of NRHM. However, in 2013, while reorganising the National Health Mission, the National Urban Health Mission (NUHM) was launched with the aim of providing affordable PHC through UPHCs, UCHCs and outreach services to the urban population in India, with special focus to people living in listed, unlisted slums, homeless, rag-pickers, migrants, and other vulnerable population [54].

The broad objectives of the IPHS for CHC in rural and urban areas include the following:

1. To define uniform benchmark ensuring high quality services that are accountable, responsive, and sensitive to the needs of the community.

2. To specify the minimum assured (Essential) and achievable (Desirable) services that are expected to be provided at CHCs in both rural and urban areas.

3. To achieve and maintain an acceptable standard of quality of care at public health facilities.

4. To facilitate monitoring and supervision of the facilities.

5. To provide guidance and tools for governance and leadership.

6. To provide guidance on health systems strengthening components which includes architectural design of facilities, human resources for health, drugs, diagnostics,

equipment, administrative and logistical support services to improve the overall health related outcomes [54].

<u>Classify the rural and urban CHC as:</u>

A. Non-FRU CHCs (rural):

Non-FRU CHCs is those that provide essential services including preventive, promotive, curative, palliative, and rehabilitative services etc. Curative services include normal delivery, stabilisation of common emergencies, etc. Non-FRU CHCs in rural areas will have 30 essential beds.

B. FRU CHCs (rural and urban):

FRU CHCs, in addition to the above services, provide specialised care which can be rendered through specialists (physicians, surgeons, obstetricians, paediatricians, and anaesthesiologists) and the accompanying infrastructure (functional operation theatre and blood storage unit). Both elective and emergency surgical services of secondary level care shall be provided. FRU-CHCs will provide surgical services and go beyond obstetric services.

Thus, while CHCs in rural areas can be either non-FRU CHC or FRU CHC, the UCHC in urban areas will function only as FRU UCHCs. Non-FRU CHCs will have 30 essential beds. For FRU CHCs in rural areas, 30 beds, maternity and surgical services will be essential while in a 50 bedded FRU CHC, additional ophthalmic, orthopaedic, and ENT services will be desirable. Similarly, for FRU UCHCs 50 beds, maternity and surgical services will be essential in all the cities. The same with 100 beds (in metropolitan cities/cities with population of more than 1 million), will have additional ophthalmic, and orthopaedic services as desirable.

The flexibility will be with the states to decide the proportion of facilities as non-FRU and FRU CHCs depending on population norms of five lakhs and/or time to care approach, availability of HR, case load and other such parameters. Likewise for urban areas, besides the above factors, the states shall have flexibility to decide the number of UCHCs depending on availability of other health facilities in the area (polyclinics, maternity homes, SDH/DH, and tertiary/medical college hospitals), to reach saturation levels as per norms.

However, since the population of urban areas varies widely, the bed requirement for UCHC shall also vary in different cities, based on the classification of non-metro or metro under the National Urban Health Mission (NUHM). Nevertheless, the number of beds at a particular UCHC is flexible and will be influenced by individual state policy taking into account the estimated facility case load, local burden of disease, access to health care and local demands.

In urban areas, following a strategic review of the 'time to care' approach and availability of other health facilities in the city/district, states should prioritise whether the existing infrastructure of UCHCs (non - functional or sub-optimally functioning) shall be utilised as such for providing secondary care or be designated as multispecialty UPHC (polyclinics) for providing assured ambulatory/day-care specialist care to the community (in case of non-feasibility of providing in-patient care and/depending on needs of the state) [54].

Block Public Health Unit (BPHU):

All CHCs at block headquarters level (in rural and urban areas) are to be developed as Block Public Health Units (BPHU). Every block in the country is envisaged as having a CHC/Block PHC/SDH at the Block Headquarter (HQ) which serves as a hub for referral from the SHCs and PHCs of the block. However, the situation across states is variable, with the Block CHC functioning as just another PHC in some states, while in some other states, the block CHC also serves as a First Referral Unit. Currently, the block health facility is only equipped to provide selected clinical services, a limited range of public health functions and administrative control of the health institutions within the block. The BPHU are expected to have four functional areas: clinical service delivery, public health functions, Block Public Health Laboratory to serve both clinical, public health functions, and HMIS unit. The clinical and diagnostic services will be delivered as per Indian Public Health Standards (IPHS) and efforts will be made to improve the quality and timeliness of reporting of service delivery and public health related data. The BPHUs will also promote decentralised planning and the preparation of block health plans that feed into district health plans [54].

Objectives:

The objectives of block public health unit will be to:

- Promote decentralized planning of public health activities with rural and urban local bodies through participatory process. District Plan will be inclusive of Block plans, Panchayat/urban local body plans.

- Serve as the referral point for the HWC- PHC and HWC-SHC in the block, in order to reduce crowding at higher level facilities, and provide comprehensive primary health care (delivery of clinical and public health services).
- Strengthen disease surveillance (both human and animal) to support evidence generation/forecast of potential outbreaks through robust data reporting using Health Management Information System (HMIS).
- To create a platform for collaboration, coordination among multi-disciplinary sectors to address social determinants of health.
- Ensure accountability for health outcomes within the block [54].

Population Norms for CHCs:

Community Health Centre in rural areas (CHC) is to be established for a population norm of 80,000 (in hilly and tribal areas) and 1,20,000 (in plains) and/or time to care approach. To establish effective convergence and linkages with citizen centric services, a CHC should be established at the Community Development Block/Taluka/Tehsil/Circle Level. This will also supplement the three-tier Panchayati System (Gram Panchayat, Block Panchayat and Zila Panchayat).

The Community Health Centre in urban areas (UCHC) is set up as a secondary care referral centre in metro cities with a population of 5 lakh and above and population of 2.5 lakh in non-metro cities. These facilities are in addition to existing facilities (SDH/DH) that cater to the urban population in the locality. A UCHC should be established at the Ward/Town/ULB/Block/City/District level to establish effective convergence and linkages with citizen centric services. It is a 50 bedded facility that provides in-patient medical, and surgical services and facilities for institutional delivery. For the metros and million plus cities, the UCHCs are established at 5 lakh population and are 100 bedded facilities.

Guidelines for Hospital Safety, 2016 – NDMA:

"Building spaces that are directly adjoining, and visible from, a main vertical evacuation route, robustly and reliably protected from heat, smoke and flame during and after a fire or any type of disaster, where people can temporarily wait with confidence for further information, instructions, and/or rescue assistance must be provisioned for. These must also be without any obstructing or interfering with the evacuation travel of other building users should also be provisioned for" [54].

Minimum performance standards for key health care staff (BPHU):

S. No.	Staff	Break up of activities
4.	Paediatrician	• OPD= 60 pts/day • IPD= 20 pts/day • 10 procedures/week
5.	Anaesthesiologist	As per the surgical requirement in OT's, in-charge and emergency services, pain clinics
6.	Ophthalmologist	• OPD= 60 pts/day • IPD= 20 pts/day • OT= 10 major surgeries/week
7.	Medical Officer	• OPD = 75 patient/day • IPD assistance with specialists • OT assistance, emergency and other duties
8.	Dentist	• OPD = 20 pts/day • Dental procedures= 8-10 (30 min./patient)
9.	Staff Nurse	As per INC norms (for OPD, IPD shifts and specialist services)
10.	Medical Laboratory Technologist/Lab technician	100 tests/day (semi-autoanalyzer), 200 tests/day (autoanalyzer)
11.	Clinical Psychologist	15-20 counselling sessions/day (30 min/per patient/day)
12.	Physiotherapist	15-20 physiotherapy intervention/day (15-20 minutes/service) Physiotherapy advice for IPD patient
13.	Social Worker	• Assess and support welfare needs (10 patient/day) • Counselling (15-20 minutes/patient) • Home visit 4/week
14.	Counsellor	20-25 counselling sessions (Group/Interpersonal)/day
15.	Dietician	• Providing dietary advice to patients, 20 patient/day • Providing nutritional and health & wellness Services • Conducting nutritional assessment • Taking anthropometric measurements • Participating in medical rounds • Record keeping

16.	ECG Technologist/ECG Technician	30-40 ECG/day technical support with TMT's
17.	OT technologist/OT Technician	Assisting in OT's, maintaining infection control practice, maintaining all equipment and instruments
18.	Radiology and Imaging Technologist/Radiology technician	X-ray: 30-40 pts/day
19.	Optometrist/Ophthalmic Assistant/Vision Technician	• 30-40 cases per day. • Detection of cataract and other basic eye ailments • Appropriate referrals • Linkages with RBSK team for refraction and issue of spectacles
20.	Dental Technician	Fabricating dental prosthetics including bridges, crowns, and dentures. Maintaining dental laboratory records. Ensuring adherence to infection prevention protocols including sterilisation.
21.	TSSU Assistant	Sterilisation services on time, packaging and labelling, pre-sterile storage, autoclaving and storage, documentation of servicing sessions
22.	Pharmacist	120 dispensations of prescription/day, maintaining stock registers, store, inventory management

SUB DISTRICT HOSPITAL & DISTRICT HOSPITAL (SDH & DH):

The delivery of services through the public health sector in India follows a three-tier structure of primary, secondary, and tertiary care services. This covers both rural and urban areas. Health system inputs (infrastructure, health workers, drugs, equipment, health information system and finances) are combined to provide quality health services that are equitable, accessible, affordable and responsive to the needs of the population. The provision of UHC forms the cornerstone for a successful public health delivery system. The High-Level Expert Group on UHC (constituted by the Government of India) defined it as "ensuring equitable access for all Indian citizens in any part of the country, regardless of income level, social status, gender, caste or religion, to affordable, accountable and appropriate, assured quality health services (promotive, preventive, curative and rehabilitative) as well as services addressing wider determinants of health delivered to individuals and populations, with the Government being the guarantor and enabler, although not necessarily the only provider of health and related services" [55]

In the year 2020, Corona Virus Infectious Disease (COVID) spread rampantly across the globe. It widely impacted health systems of countries and highlighted the need for preparing infrastructure which was resilient for responding to the need and situations brought upon by outbreaks, disease prevalence etc. This also highlighted the gaps in the availability of assured critical care and the need for a robust supply chain for the operationalisation of health facilities for timely management of critically ill patients.

To accommodate the above-mentioned changes, it was essential that a matching human resources development strategy along with an effective logistics support system and robust referral backup were duly developed. Successful implementation of these standards was to be contingent on commensurate financial support, adequate HR and an enabling public health system architecture. Previous reviews, assessments and evaluations (such as the successive Common Review Missions) demonstrated the limitations of public health facilities in meeting IPHS norms without adequate financial, HR and logistical support [55].

The broad objectives of the IPHS for public health facilities includes the following:

To define uniform benchmark ensuring high quality services that are accountable, responsive, and sensitive to the needs of the community.

1. To specify the minimum assured (Essential) and achievable (Desirable) services that are expected to be provided at different levels of public health facilities.

2. To provide guidance on health systems strengthening components which includes architectural design of facilities, human resources for health, drugs, diagnostics, equipment, administrative and logistical support services to improve the overall health related outcomes.

3. To achieve and maintain an acceptable standard of the quality of care at public facilities.

4. To facilitate monitoring and supervision of the facilities.

5. To provide guidance and tools for governance, leadership and evaluation [55].

Population Norms for SDH & DH:

The 1946 Bhore Committee report recommended one bed for every 1000 population to be increased incrementally (though several states are yet to achieve this). The National Health Policy, 2017 recommends two beds per 1000 population. It is therefore proposed that the provision of one bed per 1000 population is an 'Essential' norm for every district while two beds per 1000 is a target they should aspire towards 'Desirable'.

The 'Essential' number of beds in a district should be provided through the public health system of tertiary care (Medical Colleges), secondary care (DH, SDH and selected CHCs) and primary care (PHCs and remaining CHCs).

However, while calculating the patient-bed ratio in a district, it should primarily rely on the facilities from PHC to DH since tertiary care facilities (Medical Colleges) do not cater only to the district where it is located, but to other districts too. Care should be taken to first saturate beds at primary and secondary level public health facilities as per population norms before achieving the 'Essential' number of beds through tertiary care. To achieve the 'Desirable' number of beds, the contribution of the private sector (based on the access to private health care in the local area), Railways, Armed Forces, Power Grid, Coal fields, Employees' State Insurance (ESI) and other Public Sector Undertaking (PSU) hospitals may also be considered while continuing to strengthen and increase bed provision at public health facilities. As a thumb rule, all such beds that are available and functional for a patient for more than 24 hours, have been calculated as in-patient hospital beds (including critical care beds). The remaining beds such as

Emergency, LDR, dialysis, day-care and pre & post-operative beds have not been counted as in-patient hospital beds. However, all such beds will be counted for budgetary allocation, provision of HR, and also clinical and other support services.

- Districts with less than 5 lakh population with a functional DH do not need a Sub District hospital.
- Districts with populations between 5-10 lakh can have one SDH.

Thereafter, one SDH for every 10-lakh population can be considered for the provision of comprehensive secondary care health services [55].

Service Provision:

District hospital services have three pillars; clinical care, a knowledge hub for capacity development of HR in health, and public health programme to ensure the continuum of care and reduce the disease burden.

Clinical care includes curative, palliative, and rehabilitative services along with services for implementation of national programmes (as appropriate), provision of drugs, diagnostic services, administrative/maintenance services and other support services. Apart from curative services, there should be a strong focus on health promotion, prevention, palliation and rehabilitation at all district and Sub District hospitals.

The services to be provided at different facilities are identified as 'Essential' and 'Desirable'. The former includes those 'minimum assured services' that every facility at that level must provide. Desirable services are those that a facility should aspire to ultimately achieve (if not already being provided) over a period of time in a phased manner. 'Desirable' services indicated in the guidelines are in addition to the 'Essential' services. All infrastructure plans and human resource requirements should be based on the range of services to be provided at that facility. Critical and support services should be offered and distributed across the district in such a way that out-of-pocket expenditure (OOPE) of the community is decreased [55].

Minimum performance standards for key health care staff (SDH & DH):

Staff	Break up of activities
Staff nurse	As per INC norms (for OPD, IPD shifts and specialist services)
Medical lab technologists/Lab technician	100 tests/day (semi-autoanalyzer), 200 tests/day (autoanalyzer)
Pharmacist	120 dispensations of prescription/day, maintain stock registers, store, inventory management
Clinical Psychologist	15-20 counselling sessions/day (30 min/per patient/day)
Physiotherapist	• 15-20 physiotherapy intervention/day (15-20 minutes/service) • Physiotherapy advices for IPD patient
Medical Social Worker	• Asses and support welfare needs (5-7 patient/day) • Counselling (15-20 minutes/patient) • Home visit 4/week
Counsellor	20-25 counselling sessions/day
Dietician	• Providing dietary advice to patients, 20 patient/day • Conducting nutritional assessments • Taking anthropometric measurements • Participating in medical rounds • Record keeping
ECG technologist/technician	30-40 ECG/day, technical support with TMT's
Echo technologist/technician	Assisting in 15-20 ECHO's/day (20 min/ECHO)
OT technologist/OT technician	Assisting in OT's, maintaining infection control practice
Radiology and imaging technologist/ Radiographer	• X-ray: 30-40 pts/day (12-15 min/X-ray) • CT scan: 7-9 pts/day (40-50 min/X-ray)
Ophthalmic Assistant/Vision Technician/Optometrists	25-30 cases) for refractive assessment
Dental Technician	Fabricating dental prosthetics including bridges, crowns, and dentures. Maintain dental laboratory records

Staff	Break up of activities
Dental Hygienist	Oral prophylaxis, 15-20 procedure/day (20-25 min/pts) Record keeping
Dental Assistant	Assisting the dental surgeon with oral procedures Record keeping
Dialysis therapy technologists/ Dialysis technician	• Assisting procedures in a dialysis ward • 4 hour/patient/day (hemodialysis), 4-6 hours/patient/day (peritoneal dialysis)
Blood bank technician/Hemato Technologist	• Screening of donors • Blood collection and dispensing • Record keeping
CSSD Technician	Sterilization services on time, packaging and labeling, pre-sterile storage, autoclaving and storage, documentation of servicing sessions
Laundry technician *(for a mechanized laundry)*	• Laundry services, washing, drying, folding and ironing, sorting (critical linen for autoclaving) • Documentation of servicing session

Assuming 8 hours shift and 75% productivity and efficiency, it is estimated that there will be 6 hours of working time spread over 6 days in a week.

- Assuming an 8-hour shift and 75% of productivity and efficiency, it is estimated that there will be 6 hour working time for 6 days a week.
- Both surgical and medical specialist are expected to conduct IPD rounds every day.
- If a doctor is nominated as the nodal officer for a National Health Programme, one day per week may be dedicated to provide support to that programme (Administrative duties, monitoring, training, supervision etc. This could also be spread out on a day-to-day basis (e.g., 2 hours/day for national programme work).
- It is assumed that each surgical specialist would be having 3 OPD days and 3 OT days each week. Each surgical specialist is expected to perform at least 7 major surgeries in a week. For medical specialist with no OT duties, the OPD will be all days in a

week. Both medical and surgical specialist are expected to make IPD rounds every day.

- One GDMO for each specialist has been proposed to strengthen the service delivery and also to support the specialist in teaching and training. These GDMOs will work only in that speciality for which they are hired for [55].

HEALTH COMMITTEES:

Though all Committees have contributed towards improving health services delivery in India, the reports of the Bhore Committee, Mudaliar Committee, Jain Committee, Kartar Singh Committee, Srivastava Committee, Sidhu Committee, and Bajaj Committee will continue to guide the national health policy. The era of scientific planning in India started with the establishment of the Planning Commission in 1950. Health is fundamental to national progress. Health programmes contribute directly to the socio-economic growth of the nation. The Government of India has, therefore, been giving due attention to health in its Five-Year Plans, which has led to considerable improvement in the health of its people. There has been progressive increase in the outlay of health plans since 1950–1 till date (Ninth Plan: 1998–2002). Through the plans, specific programmes were formulated, health care institutions were built, health professionals were trained, logistics were provided, etc. Though health is largely the responsibility of states, the Central Government is responsible for higher education, research, and national health programmes, for example, family welfare, primary health care; and prevention, control, and eradication of major diseases which form the main plank of development efforts. Apart from these, the Union Ministry of Health also takes special care for preventing the spread of diseases assuming the dimension of epidemic. In addition to the schemes sponsored by the Centre, the Ministry has various World Bank sponsored projects such as District Health System Projects and control of various diseases such as AIDS, tuberculosis, malaria, blindness, and leprosy, which are implemented through the states. The Centre organizes facilities for health care of its employees and pensioners living in the capital and other major cities through Central Government Health Scheme and public hospitals. The health of the people is not only a desirable goal, but is also an essential investment in human resources. The National Health Policy (1983) reiterated India's commitment to attain HFA by the year 2000. Primary Health Care has been accepted as the key to achieve this objective. The National Health Policy affirmed that the effective delivery of health care services depends largely on the nature of education, training, and appropriate orientation towards community health of health professionals. It is imperative that the entire basis and priorities are reviewed and medical education restructured accordingly [56]

NATIONAL RURAL HEALTH MISSION: STRENGTHENING OF RURAL PUBLIC HEALTH SYSTEM:

NRHM, launched in 2005, was a watershed for the health sector in India. With its core focus to reduce maternal and child mortality, it aimed at increased public expenditure on health care, decreased inequity, decentralization and community participation in operationalization of health-care facilities based on IPHS norms. It was also an articulation of the commitment of the government to raise public spending on health from 0.9% to 2-3% of GDP. Seeking to improve access of rural people, especially poor women and children, to equitable, affordable, accountable and effective primary health care, NRHM (2005-2012) aimed to provide effective health care to the rural population throughout the country with special focus on 18 states having weak public health indicators and/or weak infrastructure. Within the mission there are high-focused and low-focused states and districts based on the status of infant and maternal mortality rates, and these states are provided additional support, both financially and technically. Gradually it has emerged as a major financing and health sector reform strategy to strengthen the state health systems. Major initiatives have been undertaken under NRHM for architectural correction of the rural health system—in terms of infrastructure, community participation, financing health care and use of information technology. Some of these activities are tabulated below. The mission emphasized on increasing health-care delivery points as well as facilities available at the health-care delivery points. It not only focused on increasing the number of physicians, specialists, staff nurses, as well as ANMs, but also gave importance to increasing the production capacity of medical colleges at graduate and post graduate levels. Physical infrastructure was enhanced by creating more health centres, new-born care units and renovating existing centres, which increased the capacity of health systems to treat more mothers and children. Special efforts were made to strengthen community participation through the formation of health committees at the village level and patient welfare committees at public health-care facilities. Information technology was used to track delivery of services to the mother and child. And all this has been an outcome of increased financial assistance by the central government and increased rates of utilization. During the period 2005-2013, the total investment by the central government equalled nearly 17 billion USD [57].

Innovation in Healthcare Delivery Systems [58]:

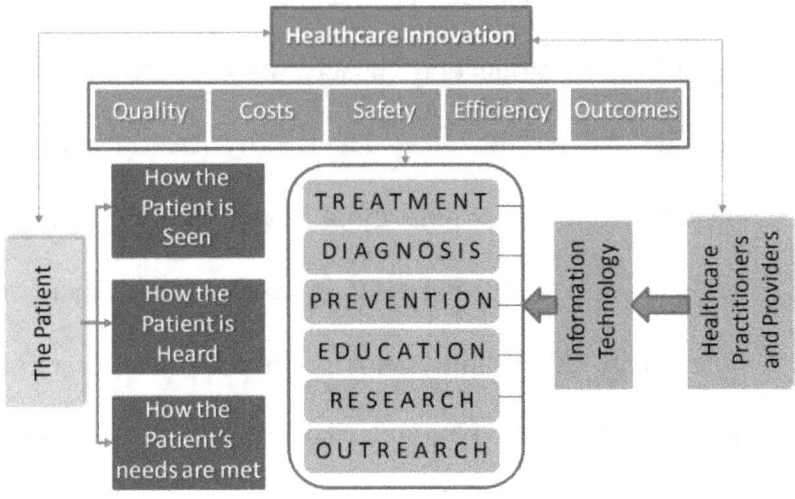

The healthcare industry has experienced a proliferation of innovations aimed at enhancing life expectancy, quality of life, diagnostic and treatment options, as well as the efficiency and cost effectiveness of the healthcare system. Information technology has played a vital role in the innovation of healthcare systems. Despite the surge in innovation, theoretical research on the art and science of healthcare innovation has been limited. One of the driving forces in research is a conceptual framework that provides researchers with the foundation upon which their studies are built [58].

SECTION 2

1. ORAL HEALTH CARE DELIVERY

Healthcare systems are responsible for addressing the needs of respective populations without any discrimination. Estimates from Global Burden of Disease demonstrate that oral diseases affect 3.9 billion people and untreated dental caries (tooth decay) is the most prevalent morbid condition among all diseases Furthermore, oral diseases significantly affect quality of life and its associated healthcare has a catastrophic effect on the public health budgets. Linkages between many oral diseases and chronic non communicable diseases are well documented and tooth loss has been reported of being associated with pre-mature mortality [59]. A good oral health reflects an aesthetic and functional dentition which allows individuals to continue in their desired social and functional role. Poor oral health leads to altered Oro-facial form and function i.e., difficulty in speaking or mastication etc. Hence the social wellbeing of an individual or the quality of life is hampered either directly or indirectly e.g., feeling ashamed of smiling in public due to crooked teeth [60].

Common oral diseases like dental caries, periodontal disease, and oral cancer satisfy the criteria for being considered as a public health problem. Evidence suggests that oral diseases share common risk factors with many other chronic diseases/ conditions such as cardiovascular diseases, diabetes, obesity, transient ischemic attacks, etc. The burden of oral diseases is high in both developed and developing nations [61].

2. ORAL HEALTH CARE DELIVERY IN DEVELOPED COUNTRIES

Oral health care systems vary from country to country and within country in terms of structure and scope, and they are directly influenced by the same factors affecting general health systems. The situation maybe further complicated by a lack of importance given to oral health and, consequently, the relationship with general health and well-being is not given the attention it deserves. Such a situation has serious implications for the type of services provided, priority of funding, program sustainability and population age groups to be served. In developing countries, data on oral diseases are scarce because of either limited economic resources or the absence of trained investigators. The basis for the scope of oral health systems may be research conducted in other countries that does not accurately represent the conditions of the developing country. It is unfortunate that the low priority given to oral health hinders the acquisition of data and the establishment of effective periodontal care programs in developing countries, but the periodontal profile is also less than satisfactory in some developed countries. There may be many reasons such low priority, including non-existent oral health policies, absence or low commitment of third-party payers, negative attitudes of oral health professionals, absence or lack of interest and ignorance on the part of the patients about predisposing risk factors, poor oral hygiene, cultural beliefs and health care traditions [62].

Oral health conditions:

Most oral health conditions are largely preventable and can be treated in their early stages. The majority of cases are dental caries (tooth decay), periodontal diseases, oral cancers, oro-dental trauma, cleft lip and palate, and noma (severe gangrenous disease starting in the mouth mostly affecting children).

The *Global Burden of Disease Study 2019* estimated that oral diseases affect close to 3.5 billion people worldwide, with caries of permanent teeth being the most common condition. Globally, it is estimated that 2 billion people suffer from caries of permanent teeth and 520 million children suffer from caries of primary teeth.

In most low- and middle-income countries, the prevalence of oral diseases continues to increase with growing urbanization and changes in living conditions. This is primarily due to inadequate exposure to fluoride (in the water supply and oral hygiene products such as toothpaste), availability and affordability of food with high sugar content and poor access to oral health care services in the community. Marketing of food and beverages high in sugar, as well as tobacco and alcohol, have led to a growing consumption of products that contribute to oral health conditions and other noncommunicable diseases [63].

Estimated global prevalence of untreated dental caries in permanent teeth [64]:

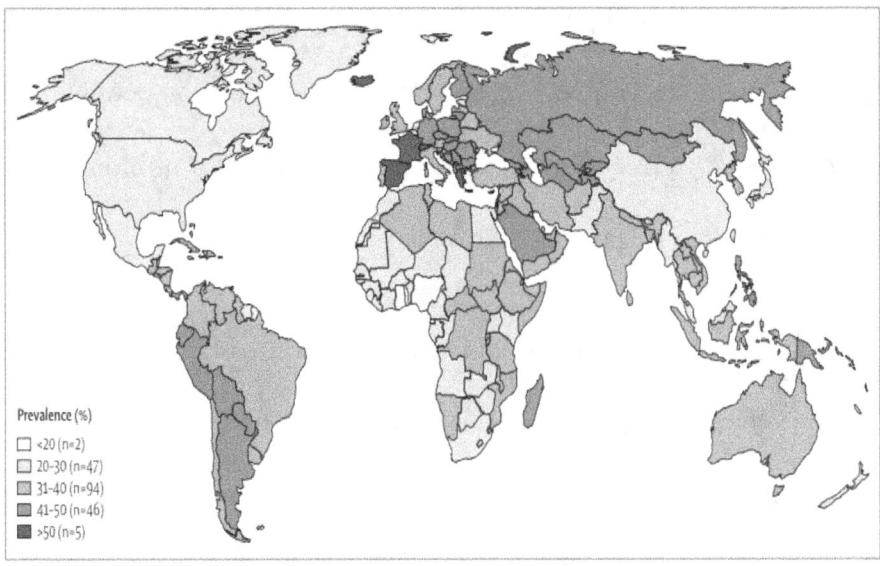

Fig; Estimated global prevalence of untreated dental caries in permanent teeth for 2017 Shown are updated age-standardised GBD estimates for 2017, obtained and visualised via the Institute of Health Metrics and

Evaluation GBD Compare tool. GBD=Global Burden of Disease. n=number of countries.

There is a strong association between oral diseases and poverty. According to the World Health Organization, oral diseases impact approximately 3.5 billion people. In addition, it is estimated that 3.9 billion people worldwide suffer from dental decay, which can impact their overall "health and well-being" and increase the burden of health care costs for already impoverished people. Many remote and underserved communities lack access to treatment and preventative services; however, several non-profits are working to increase access to dental health services globally [65].

7 NGOs Making Strides in Improving Global Dental Health:

Academy of Dentistry International Foundation. The Academy of Dentistry International is an honor society "for dentists dedicated to sharing knowledge… to serve dental health needs and to improve the quality of life throughout the world." Its Academy of Dentistry International Foundation provides grants for missions and projects that assist disadvantaged communities, supporting dental care for people in Honduras, Columbia, Kenya, Jamaica, the Philippines and Belize since 2010. The Foundation funded Bright Smiles Cameroon in 2018, which offers oral health education to school-aged children. Another grant recipient was the Health and Development Society Nepal, which offers oral health training to primary care workers who can then offer health care services to marginalized communities in Nepal.

Dentaid:

This organization began its work in 1996, delivering dental treatment to more than 70 countries since then, including the U.K. Dentaid supplies dental equipment and sends volunteers to impoverished and rural communities. Its

"DentaidBox," an innovative portable bin, includes all the equipment necessary to perform dental surgery even when electricity and running water are unavailable. In 2021, the DentaidBox reached seven African countries. In that same year, Dentaid created eight free clinics for people who are homeless in the U.K. and has plans to launch nine more. It also offered services to refugees and asylum seekers in the U.K.

Global Child Dental Fund:

This organization aims to serve every child needing dental health services. Currently, the organization is working with Jordanian dental students to aid Syrian refugees in Jordan. About 1,500 children in Jordan's refugee camps have received "toothbrushes, toothpaste and oral health education." One of the fund's projects, SEAL Cambodia, has treated more than "66,000 children with dental sealants." Global Child Dental Fund also provides "special care dentistry" in poverty-stricken and remote areas. The fund has trained students in Zambia and offered services to children with special needs in Kenya and Cambodia.

Global Dental Relief:

Since 2001, Global Dental Relief has offered free dental care to children across the world, serving close to 200,000 children from 2001 to 2020 with its volunteer work in eight countries. In addition to providing dental care, Global Dental Relief is unique in that, in Guatemala and Nepal, it also provides meals to families suffering from food scarcity.

Open Wide Foundation:

The Foundation's mission is "to bring lasting change to the state of oral health in underserved communities worldwide." The Foundation targets communities that have the greatest need for dental health care, beginning in 2012 and since serving more than 200,000 people. Open Wide Foundation built its first clinic in the Guatemalan city of Peronia, an impoverished community that had little to no access to dental health services. Since then, the Foundation has opened additional dental clinics in Guatemala. The Open Wide Foundation also works with students, offering "mentoring and practicum opportunities" to first-year dental students.

Smiles for Everyone:

Smiles for Everyone offers free dental health services in several countries. Since its inception, more than 27,000 individuals have received free dental care. Smiles for Everyone offers basic dental services as well as root canals, dentures and implants. The organization also provides training to Paraguayan dentists on complex dental procedures. Many of the patients at the free dental clinics have never visited a dentist before.

World Health Dental Organization:

This organization offers free dental care and education to marginalized communities, primarily in Kenya. Its flagship clinic provides annual dental treatment to around 4,000 Maasai people who have limited access to dental services. One particular Maasai initiative is the Momma Baby Clinic program that offers "preventative oral health and early intervention strategies... to pregnant mothers and mothers of infants and young children," educating "hundreds of mothers" a year. Another program, I Am Responsible, has led to the oral health education of more than 700 school children. The organization, through its programs, has also distributed 1,500 bamboo toothbrushes to children living in the Mara [65].

3. ORAL HEALTH CARE DELIVERY IN INDIA

Indian healthcare is organized into a three-tier system catering to primary, secondary, and tertiary levels of care. In the majority of countries across the world including India, the oral health care system has essentially been a sub-specialty of medicine rather than a unique or separate entity [61].

India is a developing country with a population of 1.21 billion. 70% of the Indian population resides in rural areas with little health care facilities and the major share of health facilities is taken up by the urban 30% population. Even in urban areas, the urban poor is a neglected lot in terms of health and oral health. Thus, there exists a huge oral health inequality among the masses in rural population [66].

Oral diseases may also impact social and psychological wellbeing, consequently leading to social isolation. The lack of regular national surveillance of oral diseases in India limits estimation of the current prevalence and the study of the trends of oral diseases. However, considering the strength of evidence on sugar intake and dental caries, and the increasing sugar intake as a consequence of rapid urbanization and subsequent westernization of diet, epidemic proportions of dental caries can be predicted in near future [59].

Furthermore, India is called as the "oral cancer capital" of the world attributed to its high intake of both smoked and smokeless tobacco products, strongly associated with oral neoplasms. Most of these highly prevalent oral diseases are largely preventable as they share common risk factors (tobacco, alcohol, unhealthy diet) with other life-threatening chronic diseases which can be reduced through various health promotion and preventive measures [59].

Vision:

All the people of India enjoy the highest possible level of dental and Oro-facial health, through promotive, preventive, curative and rehabilitative services with the highest professional standards, integrity, safety, equity and ethics [60].

Objectives

1. To strengthen oral healthcare delivery system at all levels to render promotive, preventive, curative and rehabilitative services.

2. To promote support for generating evidences, innovations, and implementation of oral health policy to control and reduce the risk factors and prevent oral diseases.

3. To encourage policy driven research, education, implementation and monitoring.

4. To build the capacity of service providers and also public health facilities for availability of skilled oral health care professionals and provision of essential oral health care services.

5. To ensure integration of oral health in all policies in multi- sectional domains including national programs under Health, Education, Work and community related policies.

6. To identify the Centers of excellence at National, Regional and State levels for generating research innovations and evidences to strengthen oral health program in the country

7. To support Centers of excellence in various activities including capacity building of service providers in the states.

8. To ensure regular monitoring and periodic evaluation of oral health program for improving the implementation and outcome envisaged under NOHP.

9. To delineate roles and responsibilities at each level (national, state and regional levels) and develop achievable targets with defined oral health outcome measures at each level.

Specific Quantitative Targets:

The policy's target is to develop robust and evidence-based outcome measures which will be defined to be collected at various levels of health care delivery systems which will form part of National Oral Health Strategic Plan document, which will be frequently reviewed and updated.

Oral Health Status

1. Establish baseline data for oral disease burden of the country by2025.

2. Reduce the morbidity and mortality from dental and oro-facial diseases by 15% by2030

Health System Performance

1. Increase utilization of public oral health facilities by at least 50% per district by2030.

2. Increase the coverage of community - based awareness programs and procedures for oral health through health care facilities by 50% by 2025; and 70% by2030

Oral Health System strengthening

Make available assured and appropriate preventive and promotive oral health services at each health & wellness center and primary health center by 2025 and in addition, make available assured curative oral health services at each Primary Health Center by 2030.

Oral Health Management Information

a. Ensure district-level electronic database of information on health system components by2025.

b. Establish integrated oral health information architecture & exchanges between district & primary health centres by2030 [60].

Oral health care in India is delivered mainly by the following establishments;

S.no	Government organizations	Private practitioners
1.	Government Dental Colleges	Private dental practitioners
2.	Government Medical Colleges and Dental Wing	Private Dental Colleges and Private dental hospitals
3.	District Hospitals with Dental Unit	Private medical hospitals with dental units.
4.	Community Health Centres	Corporate Hospitals with Dental Units.
5.	Employees State	Private Medical Colleges

	Insurance (ESI)	with Dental Wing

NATIONAL ORAL HEALTH POLICY IN INDIA:

Oral health policy in India, formulated way back, is a bleak picture even today. In 1984, national workshops were organized in Bombay on oral health targets for India and in the year 1986, oral health policy was conscripted by Indian Dental Association (IDA). Based on the recommendation of IDA, 2 more national workshops were organized, one at Delhi in 1991 and the other at Mysore after 3 years. Through the input of these 2 workshops, national oral health policy has been developed by Dental Council of India (DCI). It is the same time when World Health

Organization (WHO) had given importance to dental health by selecting the theme "Oral Health for Healthy life" for global health for the year 1994. In continuum of this, the core committee appointed by Ministry of Health and Family Welfare, GOI accepted in principle national oral health policy as a component of NHP and moved a 10-point resolution in its fourth conference in the year 1995. After 3 years, National Oral Health Care Program (NOHCP), a project of Directorate General of Health Services (DGHS) and Ministry of Health and Family Welfare was initiated and launched on a pilot basis. Later the Department of Oral and Maxillofacial Surgery, All India Institute of Medical Sciences (AIIMS) was given the charge to execute it. NOHCP, initiated as a "Pilot Project" in 5 states (Delhi, Punjab, Maharashtra, Kerala, and North Eastern states), in the process of achieving the goals of national oral health policy. Single district from each above-mentioned were selected to trial the strategies generated through 2 national and 4 regional workshops held in collaboration with AIIMS, New Delhi, in different areas of the country. The strategies of this program include oral health education with information, education and communication (IEC) materials by involving health workers, school children, teachers and mass media, formulation of basic package on rural healthcare, man power and infrastructure development, mobile dental clinic services for rural people, public health as well as research monitoring. Proposed plan for this program is depicted.

Proposed Plan for Oral Healthcare Program:

Oral Health Education	Preventive Programs	Curative Service Programs
• Training of the trainers	• Promotion of fluoride tooth paste	• Oral healthcare setup
• Oral health education chapters in school curriculum	• Legislation against tobacco products	• School dental health programs
• Oral health education through mass media	• Manufacture of sugar free chewing gums	• Manpower requirement
	• Sugar substitutes in medicinal syrups	• Equipment requirement

The project was reviewed by the National Institute of Health and Family Welfare in 2004 [67].

An Ecological Model to Advance Oral Health Equity:

Ecological models posit that factors at multiple levels influence disparities in access to and quality of services. Interventions that address factors at multiple levels may be more effective than those that target a single level. Originated in a health promotion framework by the senior author that considers dynamic social processes through which social and environmental inequalities—and associated health disparities— are produced, reproduced, and potentially transformed. It was adapted from a multilevel model of influences on oral health and health disparities that highlighted family and social factors, also by the senior author, with important contributions from the World Health Organization (WHO) concept of a health promoting school toward realizing the goal of oral health equity [68].

An Ecological Model to Advance Oral Health Equity:

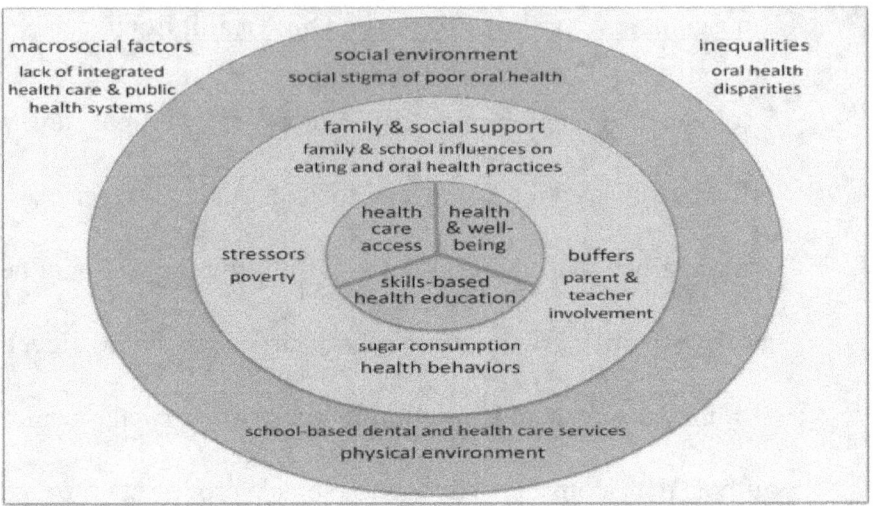

At the centre of the ecological model are the 3 outcomes of interest potentially brought about by school-based oral health programs. First, school-based oral health programs may improve health care access, as schools are often the most efficient means of providing both preventive and treatment services for children, especially for students from disadvantaged communities and families. Second, school-based oral health programs may improve general health and well-being, since oral health is fundamental to general health and has a well-documented impact on quality of life. Third, school-based oral health programs may improve skills-based health education, e.g., by enhancing understanding among students, teachers, and parents of factors that influence health, thus enabling them to make healthy choices and adopt healthy behaviours throughout their lives [69-70].

The next concentric circle in includes individual and interpersonal factors that affect these outcomes. Included therein are health behaviours, e.g., sugar consumption, as well as family and social support, e.g., influences on eating and oral health practices such as supervised toothbrushing with fluoride toothpaste, often constrained by socioeconomic conditions at home and school.

The last concentric circle in represents determinants of health- and education-related outcomes at the community level. Health promotion strategies that integrate elements of policy development and social and physical environmental factors may be yet more effective for oral disease prevention than isolated behaviour-specific interventions [68].

Policy components: [60]

Ensure Adequate Investment	The National Health Policy, 2017 has proposed to raise public health expenditure to 2.5% of the Gross Domestic Product in a time bound manner.
Comprehensive Oral Health Care (Promotive, Preventive, Curative and Rehabilitative)	Greater emphasis on promotive and preventive measures like promoting healthy eating pregnant women, preventing habits, tobacco/alcohol abuse, preventive care and oral health education in Information Education Communication/Behaviour Change Communication, oral

	health screening programs, tooth dental clean brushing activities in school, professional dental cleaning, fluoride varnish application and pit and fissure sealant programs.
Accessible and Affordable Oral Healthcare	Special focus on rural, hard to reach and tribal areas to improve access to accountable, primary oral health care services in line with the universal health coverage philosophy
Quality of Life	To establish an oral health promoting environment conducive to lead a quality life. To provide appropriate preventive and promotive measures pertaining to oral diseases

Integration	Relevant National Health Programs
	Inter-Ministerial Collaborations
	Educational Institutions
Community involvement	Community leaders, Panchayati Raj Institutions, Self Help Groups and civil society
Partnership	Private sector, preferably from not-for-profit organizations, for an efficient oral health care delivery and to strengthen preventive and promotive oral health activities.
Common Risk Factor Approach (CRFA)	Consorted efforts aligning with other noncommunicable disease control policies by using Common Risk Factor Approach as a major strategy.
Information	To augment mass awareness on

Education Communication/ Behaviour Change Communication	dental and oral diseases, prevention and healthy practices using available contemporary modalities in local/ regional context, with special emphasis on high risk and vulnerable populations.
Patient cantered quality of life	The need for public and private health facilities rendering oral health care services to cater patient friendly, need based, and evidence based, quality care, acceptable to the patient, considering cultural and social factors.
Health System Strengthening	Oral health care personnel at all levels of health care delivery and support systems of the country.
Accountability,	Recommends the use of

Monitoring and Evaluation	performance indicators to assess output and outcomes of the system. It looks to establishing a central site for aggregating survey results and developing a robust Health Management Information System
Oral health research	The areas of research may include fundamental dental research, epidemiological, operational and implementation research of national importance. It supports the establishment of Centres of Oral Health Research across India
Dental education	To strengthen the quality of higher education in all specialties of dentistry with focus on overall health promotion and promote

	teaching, research and innovation at all levels of dental education.
Advocacy	Advocacy at all levels of governance is required for increased political and financial commitment for oral health.

4. ORAL HEALTH CARE INSURANCE IN INDIA

With the advent of the 21st century and the stability in the Indian economy, the dental insurance prospect of business remains unexplored. The Government of India and its policies are to be blamed for this sector to be left out. Due to the large population of the country, insurance sector needs foreign collaboration in order to cover all aspects of insurance. The Foreign Direct Investment (FDI) bill which was put forward in the winter session of the parliament (2008) focused on increasing the FDI investment share from 26% to 49% [71].

Health insurance schemes such as the employee's state insurance scheme and Central Government health scheme which provides for comprehensive medical care along with optical and dental aids at reasonable rates.[72]

The current budget allocation (Budget Estimate or BE) in the current year 2022-23 is Rs 86,200.65 crore which is a 16.59 per cent increase compared to the BE of Rs 73,931.77 crore in 2021-22. However, if the revised estimate (RE) budget for the year 2021-22 which was Rs 86,000.65 is compared, the allocation to the health ministry is barely 0.23 per cent. The National Health Policy 2017 envisages increasing the public health expenditure to 2.5 per cent of the GDP by 2025. India also doesn't seem to be reaching that target with the pace of the increments in the health budget. "India is among the top 10 countries in the world incurring a very high magnitude of out-of-pocket expenditure. On the other hand, India also faces the challenge of housing a very high proportion of households with low incomes. In such situations India should be spending at least 2.5 per cent of GDP on health sector, as suggested by the National Health Policy of India way back in 2017 [73].

Oral health's are not integrated with the general health insurance schemes. The efforts of the Indian Dental Association to bring out a comprehensive Indian dental insurance scheme have seen partial success so far. Indian dental insurance plans are mainly of two types: Stand-alone dental insurance plan: This type of plan covers the expenses related to general dental problems such as periodontitis and extraction of permanent teeth due to ailments such as caries. The amount of expense to be reimbursed as well as the period of such cover is fixed. This type of plan is generally provided by the popular dental care product companies in association with one of the insurance companies. The first of its kind dental insurance scheme in India was launched through oral care brand, Pepsodent in 2002. This plan was in partnership with the New India Assurance; the plan offered a dental insurance of Rs. 1000 on purchase of any pack of Pepsodent. Insurance cover against expenses for the extraction of teeth due to caries and periodontitis was also provided. But this plan was time bound and also did not cover other aspects of dental rehabilitation [71].

Indian Dental Association has been striving to bring out a new all-inclusive oral and dental health care insurance scheme. However, it has been unable to achieve anything substantial in this front. We, as oral health care workers, are capable to reach every class and village across the country.

Dental health insurance can also bring about dental health care awareness percolating at the gross root levels. It would serve as a good motivation to the people to regularly visit the dentist and this in turn serves as an effective preventive measure. If we have to create the awareness and pass on the benefits of longevity of teeth across the society, dental profession should impress on to the policy makers to have beneficial dental insurance schemes for the masses.[71]

Health insurances must persuade the coverage of dental treatments. Employees' State Insurance (ESI), 1948 is such a scheme by the Indian government which includes dental health. It was recommended that insurance companies or any other independent agents should not be allowed to procure medical services on behalf of the public sector. India should come up with schemes like unified health system, 1988 in Brazil, National Health Insurance (NHI), 1995 in Taiwan, Social Health Insurance (SHI) in Germany and National Social Health Insurance Fund (NSHIF), 2004 in Kenya, that covers oral procedures under hospital care.[74]

Improving oral health means improving general health and well-being of the community and in essence it is improving the quality of life and developing healthy life styles (brushing, eating protective foods, avoiding smoking and Pan chewing etc.) in children, adolescents, adults and senior citizens. NOHCP is a multi-sector endeavour, leadership of dentists is essential to sustain the activities. The leadership is required to effectively coordinate the functions of school health activities, non-formal educators, ICDS Anganwadis, water and sanitation programme, Nutrition Policy, health workers Primary Health Care Sector, food adulteration, popular mass media, and national cancer control programme, and above all the communities, homes and parents as also Panchayati Raj Institutions (PRI) to achieve the desired goals. Convergence of services of different sectors is essential to mitigate the dental problems (dental decay, periodontal disease, oral cancers and malocclusion) [75].

SECTION – 3

HEALTH INSURANCE

Health insurance is one of the important approaches that can help in boosting Universal Health Coverage (UHC) through improved healthcare utilisation and financial protection. There are multiple types of insurance in Low-income and middle-income countries (LMICs) that differ with providers (government vs private sector), scales and types of beneficiaries [76].

Health insurance literacy is defined as 'the degree to which individuals have the knowledge, ability and confidence to find and evaluate information about health plans, select the best plan for their own (or their families) financial and health circumstances, and use the plan once enrolled.' Lack of health insurance literacy or education hinders the uptake of health insurance and in many Low-income and middle-income countries (LMICs) health insurance literacy is poor. A study conducted in Uganda reported that about 34% of the studied population were not aware of health insurance. LMICs contribute to around 84% of the world population and 90% of the global burden of disease [59].

People living in the LMICs rely majorly on out-of-pocket payments as the prime source for managing healthcare expenses, that results in a massive demand for services and financial burden of households (usually catastrophic), which in turn leads to impoverishment. It is projected that every year approximately 150 million people experience financial catastrophe, by spending more than 40% on health expenses other than food. Families generally spend more than 10% of the household income on illness-related expenses, due to which other household expenses are affected. To make it worse, evidence suggests that per capita spending on healthcare in many LMICs is expected to increase in coming years. Additionally, the increased costs of seeking and receiving care can hinder the access to healthcare [76].

The Universal Health Coverage (UHC) is embedded within the Sustainable Development Goals (SDGs) and aims 'to ensure healthy lives and promote well-being for all at all ages by 2030'. It includes financial risk protection and equal access to quality essential healthcare services [78].

In other terms, UHC encourages equitable healthcare and nations across the world are committed to achieving SDGs through UHC [79].

HEALTH INSURANCE IN INDIA:

India's first health insurance programme, launched in the 1950s, was limited to central government employees and certain low-income population. Over the years, the private healthcare providers' dominance in quality healthcare service provision can be seen. Nevertheless, many economically backward families are either deprived of healthcare or are pushed into poverty in the absence of financial protection. In 2002, targeted health insurance programmes for low-income households were introduced by central and state governments in partnership with private sector and non-governmental organisations (NGO). Since 2002 (recommendations of National Health Policy 2002), more than 17 health insurance schemes have been launched by various governments in India [80]

There is no universal health insurance in India. Health insurance is at present limited to industrial workers and their families. The Central Government employees are also covered by the health insurance, under the banner "Central Govt. Health Scheme" [5].

Employees State Insurance Scheme:

The ESI scheme, introduced by an Act of Parliament in 1948, is a unique piece of social legislation in India. It has introduced for the first time in India the principle of contribution by the employer and employee. The Act provides for medical care in cash and kind, benefits in the contingency of sickness, maternity, employment injury, and pension for dependents on the death of worker because of employment injury. The Act covers employees drawing wages not exceeding Rs. 15,000 per month.

Central Government Health Scheme:

The Central Government Health Scheme (previously known as Contributory Health Service Scheme) for the Central Government employees was first introduced in New Delhi in 1954 to provide comprehensive medical care to Central Government employees. The scheme is based on the principle of cooperative effort by the employee and the employer, to the mutual advantage of both.

The facilities under the scheme include:

(a) out-patient care through a network of dispensaries

(b) supply of necessary drugs

(c) laboratory and X-ray investigations

(d) domiciliary visits

(e) hospitalization facilities at Government as well as private hospitals recognized for the purpose

(f) specialist consultation

(g) paediatric services including immunization

(h) antenatal, natal and postnatal services

(i) emergency treatment

(j) supply of optical and dental aids at reasonable rate, and

(k) family welfare services [5].

The scope of the scheme has been gradually extended over the years to cover cities outside Delhi as well as other sectors of population such as the employees of the autonomous organizations, retired Central Govt, servants, widows receiving family pension, Members of Parliament, Ex-Governors and retired Judges. The Scheme now covers besides Delhi, the cities of Mumbai, Allahabad, Meerut, Kanpur, Patna, Kolkata, Nagpur, Chennai, Hyderabad, Bangalore, Jaipur, Pune, Lucknow, Ahmedabad, Bhubaneshwar, and Jabalpur.

The scheme which started with 16 allopathic dispensaries in 1954 covering 2.3 lakh beneficiaries has now 320 dispensaries/hospitals in various systems of medicine and provides service to about 42.76 lakh beneficiaries. There is also a yoga centre under the scheme in Delhi.

The Employees State Insurance Scheme and the Central Government Health Scheme cover two large groups of wage-earners in the country. They are well-organized health insurance schemes, and are providing reasonable medical care plus some essential preventive and promotive health services. Experience in other countries has shown that health insurance is a logical step towards nationalization of health services [5].

The most recent one is 'Ayushman Bharat' or Pradhan Mantri Jan Arogya Yojana (PMJAY) (Prime minister's health assurance scheme) launched in 2018 to achieve UHC. PMJAY is fully financed by the government and seeks to cover 500million citizens with an annual cover of approximately US$7000 per household. The main aim of the PMJAY is to lessen the economic burden experienced by poor and vulnerable groups for access to healthcare facility [81].

CONCLUSION:

Even though India has created one of the largest health care delivery systems in the world, people of country still suffer from a multitude of preventable and treatable general and oral health problems. Opportunities exists to integrate oral health care with general health care, but weak political will, less patient awareness and economic factors restricts this noble idea. Attempts should be made to improve the quality of life of the population through research, education, provision of services, and through the promotion of healthy policies.

In nutshell oral health care systems includes

1. Health policies to promote Oral Health,

2. Resources including personnel and facilities,

3. Strategies that organizes those resources to provide services.

In order to improve a system within a country, it is important to gain knowledge from systems internationally [82].

REFERENCE:

1. Healthcaredeliverytranscript.www.coursehero.com/file/58114254/healthcaredeliverytranscriptpdf/ Accessed on: 09/03/2022.

2. Hasan MZ, Singh S, Arora D, Jain N, Gupta S. Evidence of integrated primary-secondary health

care in low-and middle-income countries: protocol for a scoping review. Systematic reviews. 2020 Dec;9(1):1-8.

3. Bernstein AB. Health care in America: trends in utilization. Center for Disease Control and Prevention, National Center for Health Statistics; 2004.

4. Sharma DA. Indian health groups demand right to health. Lancet 2004; 363:1044

5. Park k textbook of preventive and social medicine. 26th edition, 2021.

6. Kandelman D, Arpin S, Baez RJ, Baehni PC, Petersen PE. Oral health care systems in developing and developed countries. Periodontology 2000. 2012 Oct;60(1):98-109.

7. Younger DS. Health care in India. Neurologic clinics. 2016 Nov 1;34(4):1103-14.

8. Kasthuri A. Challenges to healthcare in India-the five A's. Indian journal of community medicine: official publication of Indian Association of Preventive & Social Medicine. 2018 Jul;43(3):141.

9. Satpathy SK. Indian public health standards (IPHS) for community health centres. Indian J Public Health. 2005 Jul 1;49(3):123-6.

10. Tabish SA. Historical Development of Health Care in India. Research gate. 2000 Jan.

11. Camillo CA. The US healthcare system: Complex and unequal. Global Social Welfare. 2016 Sep;3(3):151-60.

12. Department for Professional Employees [Internet]. The US health care system: An international perspective.

13. OECD (2015). Health at a glance 2015: OECD indicators. Paris: OECD Publishing

14. Cockerham WC. Health Care Delivery System: Russia. The Wiley Blackwell Encyclopedia of Health, Illness, Behavior, and Society. 2014 Jan 6:842-8.

15. The healthcare system in Russia | Expatica Accessed on: 14/6/22.

16. Understanding Russia's Healthcare System and Options for Expats (internationalinsurance.com)] Accessed on: 14/6/22.

17. Yi B. An overview of the Chinese healthcare system. Hepatobiliary Surgery and Nutrition. 2021 Jan;10(1):93.

18. Data from China Banking and Insurance Regulatory Commission. Available online: http://www.cbirc.gov.cn/ cn/view/pages/index/index.html

19. Opinions on Deepening the Reform of Medical Security System, The CPC Central Committee, The

State Council. 2020. Available online: http://www.gov.cn/ zhengce/2020-03/05/content_5487407.htm

20. Healthcare in the UAE and Saudi Arabia October 2021 what's the opportunity? Access on: Healthcare report UAE and KSA 2021.cdr (ctfassets.net)

21. The state of health in the WHO African region. An analysis of the status of health, health services and health systems in the context of the Sustainable Development Goals. Access on: State of health in the African Region.pdf (who.int)

22. Health care quality in Africa: Uganda, Nigeria, Tanzania, Zambia, Kenya, Zimbabwe and South Africa. Access on: Health care quality in Africa: Uganda, Nigeria, Tanzania, Zambia, Kenya, Zimbabwe and South Africa | Aetna International

23. Laugesen K, Ludvigsson JF, Schmidt M, Gissler M, Valdimarsdottir UA, Lunde A, Sørensen HT. Nordic

health registry-based research: a review of health care systems and key registries. Clinical epidemiology. 2021; 13:533.

24. Schmidt M, Schmidt SAJ, Adelborg K, et al. The Danish health care system and epidemiological research: from health care contacts to database records. Clin Epidemiol. 2019; 11:563–591.

25. Anell A, Glenngård AH, Merkur S. Sweden health system review. Health Syst Transit. 2012;14(5):1–159.

26. 1177 Vårdguiden. Available from: https://www.1177.se/ Orebrolan/sa-fungerar-varden/varden-i-orebro-lan/egen-vardbe garan/. Accessed February 10, 2021.

27. Ludvigsson JF. The first eight months of Sweden's COVID-19 strategy and the key actions and actors that were involved. Acta Paediatrica. 2020.

28. OECD/European Observatory on Health Systems and Policies. Sweden: Country Health Profile 2017, State of Health in the EU, OECD Publishing. Brussels: Paris/European Observatory on Health Systems and Policies; 2017

29. Gaardsrud PØ. Styringsdata for fastlegeordningen. kvartal. 2019; 4:2019.

30. Sperre Saunes IKM, Sagan A. Norway: Health System Review. Health Systems in Transition. 2020.

31. Keskimäki ITL, Reissell E, Koivusalo M, et al. Finland: Health System Review. Health Systems in Transition. 2019.

32. Sigurgeirsdóttir SWJ, Maresso A. Iceland: health system review. Health System Transit. 2014;6(16):1–182.

33. The Icelandic Ministry of Health. Health Policy. A Policy for Iceland's Health Services Until 2030; 2019.

34. Sjúkratryggingar Íslands. Health Insurance in Iceland. Available at: https://www.sjukra.is/english/social-insurance-in-iceland/payment-participation-system/. Accessed April 12, 2021.

35. Sigriour Haralds Elinardottir. Director of Health Statistics, Directorade of Health, Iceland.

36. Health care quality in Southeast Asia: Singapore, Thailand, Brunei, Hong Kong, Vietnam and Indonesia.www.aetnainternational.com/en/about-us/explore/living-abroad/culture-lifestyle/health-care-quality-in-southeast-asia.html. Accessed on: 15/6/22

37. Bitton A, Ratcliffe HL, Veillard JH, Kress DH, Barkley S, Kimball M, Secci F, Wong E, Basu L, Taylor C, Bayona J. Primary health care as a foundation for strengthening health systems in low-

and middle-income countries. Journal of general internal medicine. 2017 May;32(5):566-71.

38. Primary health care (who.int) Access on: 15/4/2022

39. Hasan MZ, Singh S, Arora D, Jain N, Gupta S. Evidence of integrated primary-secondary health care in low-and middle-income countries: protocol for a scoping review. Systematic reviews. 2020 Dec;9(1):1-8.

40. Infrastructure: National Health Mission (nhm.gov.in)Health workforce: Dentistry personnel (who.int) Accessed on: 28/4/2022

41. Chokshi M, Patil B, Khanna R, Neogi SB, Sharma J, Paul VK, Zodpey S. Health systems in India. Journal of Perinatology. 2016 Dec;36(3): S9-12.

42. Hiremath SS. Textbook of preventive and community dentistry. Elsevier India; 2011 Aug 15.

43. PHC IPHS Guidelines 2022.pdf (nhm.gov.in). Accessed on: 28/03/2022

44. Universal Health in the 21st Century: 40 Years of Alma-Ata - World | Relief Web. Accessed on: 18/04/2022

45. Rifkin SB. Alma Ata after 40 years: Primary Health Care and Health for All—from consensus to complexity. BMJ global health. 2018 Dec 1;3(Suppl 3): e001188.

46. Declaration of Alma-Ata (who.int) Access on: 22/5/2022

47. Lahariya C. Health & wellness centers to strengthen primary health care in India: Concept, progress and ways forward. The Indian Journal of Pediatrics. 2020 Nov;87(11):916-29.

48. INDIAN PUBLIC HEALTH STANDARDS Health and wellness centre- sub Health centre. SHC HWC UHWC IPHS Guidelines-2022.pdf (nhm.gov.in) Access on: 25/5/2022

49. Cherian SA, Joseph E, Rupesh S, Syriac G, Philip J. Empowerment of anganwadi workers in oral health care: A Kerala experience. International Journal of Clinical Pediatric Dentistry. 2019 Jul;12(4):268.

50. GUIDELINES ON ACCREDITED SOCIAL HEALTH ACTIVITISTS (ASHA). Guidelines on ASHA.doc (nhm.gov.in) Access on: 25/5/2022

51. Press Information Bureau. Government of India. Ministry of Health and Family Welfare. ASHA Workers. ASHA Workers (pib.gov.in) Access on: 14/4/2022

52. Guidelines for Performance Incentives under POSHAN Abhiyaan. Performance Incentive Guidelines 01-11-2021.pdf (wcd.nic.in) Access on: 06/04/22.

53. Primary, Secondary and Tertiary HealthCare - Arthapedia Access on: 09/03/2022

54. INDIAN PUBLIC HEALTH STANDARDS COMMUNITY HEALTH CENTRE. CHC IPHS Guidelines-2022.pdf Access on: 25/5/2022

55. INDIAN PUBLIC HEALTH STANDARDS SUB DISTRICT HOSPITAL and DISTRICT hospital. SDH DH IPHS Guidelines-2022.pdf Access on: 25/5/2022

56. Tabish SA. Historical Development of Health Care in India. Historical Development of Health Care in India pdf Access on: 27/5/2022

57. Chokshi M, Patil B, Khanna R, Neogi SB, Sharma J, Paul VK, Zodpey S. Health systems in India. Journal of Perinatology. 2016 Dec;36(3): S9-12.

58. Omachonu VK, Einspruch NG. Innovation in healthcare delivery systems: a conceptual framework. The Innovation Journal: The Public Sector Innovation Journal. 2010 Mar 1;15(1):1-20.

59. Mathur MR, Singh A, Watt R. Addressing inequalities in oral health in India: Need for skill mix in the dental workforce. Journal of family medicine and primary care. 2015 Apr;4(2):200.

60. DRAFT NATIONAL ORAL HEALTH POLICY https://main.mohfw.gov.in/sites/default/files/N_568 20_1613385504626.pdf

61. Ramanarayanan V, Chandrasheka r Janakiram JJ, Krishnakumar K. Oral health care system analysis: A case study from India. Journal of Family Medicine and Primary Care. 2020 Apr;9(4):1950.

62. Kandelman D, Arpin S, Baez RJ, Baehni PC, Petersen PE. Oral health care systems in developing and developed countries. Periodontology 2000. 2012 Oct;60(1):98-109.

63. Oral health. https://www.who.int/news-room/fact-sheets/detail/oral-health

64. Peres MA, Macpherson LM, Weyant RJ, Daly B, Venturelli R, Mathur MR, Listl S, Celeste RK, Guarnizo-Herreño CC, Kearns C, Benzian H. Oral diseases: a global public health challenge. The Lancet. 2019 Jul 20;394(10194):249-60.

65. 7 NGOS CONTRIBUTING TO GLOBAL DENTAL HEALTH https://borgenproject.org/dental-health/

66. Singh SH, Shah VA, Dagrus KA, Manjunatha BS, Kariya PB, Shah SN. Oral health inequality and barriers to oral health care in India. European Journal of Dental Therapy and Research. 2015;4(1):242-5.

67. Kothia NR, Bommireddy VS, Devaki T, Vinnakota NR, Ravoori S, Sanikommu S, Pachava S. Assessment of the status of national oral health policy in India. International journal of health policy and management. 2015 Sep;4(9):575.

68. Gargano L, Mason MK, Northridge ME. Advancing oral health equity through school-based oral health programs: An ecological model and review. Frontiers in public health. 2019 Nov 26; 7:359.

69. Petersen PE. The World Oral Health Report 2003: continuous improvement of oral health in the 21st century-the approach of the WHO Global Oral Health Programme. Community Dent. Oral Epidemiol. (2003) 31(Suppl. 1):3– 23.

70. Kwan SYL, Petersen PE, Pine CM, Borutta A. Health-promoting schools: an opportunity for oral health promotion. Bull. World Health Org. (2005) 83:677–85.

71. Toor RS, Jindal R. Dental insurance! Are we ready? Indian Journal of Dental Research. 2011 Jan 1;22(1):144.

72. Puzhankara L, Janakiram C. Medical-dental integration-achieving equity in periodontal and

general healthcare in the Indian scenario. Journal of International Society of Preventive & Community Dentistry. 2021 Jul;11(4):359.

73. <u>Budget 2022: Despite raging pandemic, healthcare receives marginal allocation - Business Today. Access on: 29/05/2022</u>

74. Kothia NR, Bommireddy VS, Devaki T, Vinnakota NR, Ravoori S, Sanikommu S, Pachava S. Assessment of the status of national oral health policy in India. International journal of health policy and management. 2015 Sep;4(9):575.

75. Lal S, Paul D, Vashisht BM. National oral health care programme (NOHCP) implementation strategies. Indian Journal of Community Medicine. 2004 Jan 1;29(1):3.

76. Reshmi B, Unnikrishnan B, Parsekar SS, Rajwar E, Vijayamma R, Venkatesh BT. Health insurance awareness and its uptake in India: a systematic

review protocol. BMJ open. 2021 Apr 1;11(4): e043122.

77. Basaza R, Kyasiimire EP, Namyalo PK, et al. Willingness to pay for community health insurance among TAXI drivers in Kampala City, Uganda: a contingent evaluation. Risk Manag Healthc Policy 2019; 12:133–43.

78. van Hees SGM, O'Fallon T, Hofker M, et al. Leaving no one behind? social inclusion of health insurance in low- and middle-income countries: a systematic review. Int J Equity Health 2019; 18:134.

79. Fadlallah R, El-Jardali F, Hemadi N, et al. Barriers and facilitators to implementation, uptake and sustainability of community-based health insurance schemes in low- and middle-income countries: a systematic review. Int J Equity Health 2018; 17:13.

80. Maurya D, Mintrom M. Policy entrepreneurs as catalysts of broad system change: the case of social

health insurance adoption in India. J Asian Public Policy 2020; 13:18–34

81. Garg S, Bebarta KK, Tripathi N. Performance of India's national publicly funded health insurance scheme, Pradhan Mantri Jan Arogaya Yojana (PMJAY), in improving access and financial protection for hospital care: findings from household surveys in Chhattisgarh state. BMC Public Health 2020; 20:949.

82. Batra P, Saini P, Yadav V. Oral health concerns in India. Journal of Oral Biology and Craniofacial Research. 2020 Apr 1;10(2):171-4.